Chronic Pain Management

Chronic Pain Management

Edited by

CAROL BANKS MSc, RN

Basildon and Thurrock University Hospitals NHS Foundation Trust

and

KAREN MACKRODT MSc, RGN

Mid-Essex Hospital Service NHS Trust

W
WHURR PUBLISHERS
LONDON AND PHILADELPHIA

© 2005 Whurr Publishers Ltd
First published 2005
by Whurr Publishers Ltd
19b Compton Terrace
London N1 2UN England and
325 Chestnut Street, Philadelphia PA 19106 USA

Reprinted 2005

British Library Cataloguing in Publication Data

A catalogue record for this book
is available from the British Library.

ISBN 1 86156 453 8

Typeset by Adrian McLaughlin, a@microguides.net
Printed and bound in the UK by Athenæum Press Ltd, Gateshead, Tyne & Wear.

Contents

Foreword   vii
Preface   ix
Contributors   xi
Editors' note   xiii
Acknowledgements   xvii
Introduction   xix

Chapter 1 Models of health and illness   1

Annie Sheldrake

Chapter 2 Physiology of chronic pain   36

Mark Johnson

Chapter 3 Living with pain through the eyes of the sufferer   75

Karen Mackrodt

Chapter 4 Appraising pain   92

Carolyn Mackintosh

Chapter 5 Barriers to effective pain management   113

Alison Gray

Chapter 6 Invasive techniques   129

Carol Banks

Chapter 7 Psychological perspectives   155

Ruth Madeleine Dallob, Cristina López-Chertudi, Tricia Rose

Chapter 8 Reactivation   **186**

Jan Cooil

Chapter 9 Self-treatment strategies   **210**

Jan Cooil

Chapter 10 Pharmacological management   **230**

Peter Croot

Chapter 11 Complementary therapies   **258**

Val Ali

Index   271

Foreword

Healthcare exists to prolong life and to improve health-related quality of life. Governments, which are servants of the people, provide a healthcare service for the people. What is it we want this service to achieve? When you look at what we do, it becomes apparent that most of what we spend our time and money on is improving health-related quality of life.

The presence of chronic pain is one of the main variables in determining health-related quality of life. Despite this, we are not so good at directing our healthcare system to do much about it. Healthcare systems have developed into structures where the emphasis is on treatment of the underlying disease with the presumption that this will manage the presenting symptoms. When this approach (the traditional medical model) does not always work we should ask ourselves why.

A Europe-wide telephone survey in 2004 of a random but representative sample of citizens in 16 countries found that 19% of the population had experienced chronic pain for more than 6 months and had suffered it in the preceding month. The actual average duration of pain was 7 years. The most common condition was 'back pain' (24%) and the commonest cause attributed by those asked was 'arthritis' (35%). One person in five had lost his or her job due to pain and a similar number had been diagnosed with depression; 40% felt that their everyday activities had been affected by pain. There was a considerable variation of prescribing practice for pain from one country to another. Only 2% volunteered that they had been referred to a pain-management clinic (www.painineurope.com).

The prevalence of chronic pain in our community is enormous. Many of those sampled would probably benefit from quite simple medical, educational and behavioural intervention. Some might well need referral to a specialist pain management unit and others might prove relatively intractable. We need to wake up to the reality that our traditional ideas about patient and pain management are undergoing a revolution. This revolution has occurred within the pain management specialties but now, if we are to tackle pain in our society, we need understanding and commitment from all those involved in treating patients, many of whom will have unresolved persistent and intrusive pain.

Chronic Pain Management is deliberately aimed at this audience and as such will be a major contributor to patient welfare far beyond the pain-management clinic.

Simon Thomson MBBS, FRCA, FIPP
2004

Preface

Pain, and particularly chronic pain, is a debilitating and disabling condition. Persistent pain can interrupt all aspects of a person's life and every nurse will experience people who are suffering chronic pain with varied degrees of interruption to their lives. Those caring for people in pain need to be aware of the impact of chronic persistent pain on the lives of sufferers and those close to them in order to have any degree of understanding and empathy of the situation they are in.

The nature and complexity of pain create a challenge for any nurse coming into contact with a chronic pain sufferer. The nurse needs to recognize that there are many elements with equal complexities that form an indistinguishable part of the whole pain experience.

In our experience of working with chronic pain sufferers we have become aware of a gap in the literature pertaining to the nursing management of chronic pain patients. One of the inspirations for this book came from the publication of *Recommendations for Nursing Practice in Pain Management* (The Pain Society, 2002), which clearly defines the competencies required in order to underpin clinical practice with evidence-based approaches.

The aim of this book is to enable the reader to become competent in the assessment, planning and evaluation of an episode of care, while enabling the nurse to empower those experiencing chronic pain to understand their pain and ultimately to take responsibility for their own management.

It will cover many aspects of the chronic pain experience while attempting to identify the various models associated with the delivery of chronic pain techniques. It looks at the delivery of care by professionals working in both the community and hospital setting as well as looking at how those suffering pain can be involved actively in their management. However, it will only look at chronic pain management with respect to adults.

The editors have sought authors from different backgrounds – from academia as well as from health-professional arenas – thus striking a balance between theory and practice. The book has been set out with each chapter containing learning objectives. The reader can try to achieve them through reflective practice.

Chronic Pain Management will be particularly useful for final year nursing students, qualified hospital and community-based nurses, and any health professional caring for people in chronic pain.

Reference

The Pain Society (2002) Recommendations for Nursing Practice in Pain Management. London: The Pain Society.

Contributors

Val Ali MSc, BSc(Hons), RGN, Lic.Ac. Consultant nurse in chronic pain, East Kent Hospitals NHS Trust

Carol Banks MSC, RN, Nurse specialist, pain management, Basildon and Thurrock University Hospitals NHS Foundation Trust

Jan Cooil MSc, MCSP, SRP, Superintendent 1 physiotherapist, Thurrock Primary Care Trust

Peter Croot BPharm, MSc, MRPharms, Pharmacy manager, Basildon and Thurrock University Hospitals NHS Foundation Trust

Ruth Madeleine Dallob BSc(Hons), MSc, RGN, DN Postgraduate Diploma Counselling, Counselling psychologist, South Essex Partnership NHS Trust

Alison Gray Palliative care sister, Macmillan Team, Mid-Essex Hospital Service NHS Trust, Chelmsford, Essex

Mark Johnson BSc, PhD, School of Health Sciences, Leeds Metropolitan University

Cristina López-Chertudi BSc(Hons), MSc, CPsychol(Clin), Chartered clinical psychologist, South Essex Partnership NHS Trust

Carolyn Mackintosh PGDip(HE), MSc, BA(Hons), RGN, Senior lecturer, Division of Nursing, University of Bradford

Karen Mackrodt MSc, BSc(Hons), RGN, Nurse specialist, pain management, Mid-Essex Hospital Service NHS Trust, Chelmsford, Essex

Tricia Rose MSc Psych, Accredited counselling psychologist, South Essex Partnership NHS Trust

Annie Sheldrake PhD, Clinical psychologist, Spectrum, Chelmsford and Essex Hospital, Chelmsford, Essex

Simon Thomson MBBS, FRCA, FIPP, Consultant in pain management and anaesthesia, Basildon and Thurrock University Hospitals NHS Foundation Trust, President of UK and Ireland chapter of the International Neuromodulation Society, Secretary of the World International Neuromodulation Society

Editors' note

The aim of this book is to enhance the use of the *Recommendations for Nursing Practice in Pain Management* developed by the Nursing Focus in Pain Management working party of the Pain Society (2002).

The Pain Society competencies use core elements of Benner's (1984) work in defining a path from novice to expert. Three levels of proficiency are highlighted: novice, intermediate and higher-level practice. This book aims to provide the reader with an understanding of the nature of chronic pain and how it affects the whole construct of the patient and surrounding environment. We have therefore concentrated on the competencies developed by the working party of the British Pain Society (formerly the Pain Society) at the novice and intermediate levels.

Recommendations for nursing practice in pain management are available from the British Pain Society website: www.britishpainsociety.org.

Nursing competencies in pain management

The competencies addressed in this book are as follows.

Chapters 3, 4, 5, 7, 8, 9, 10 and 11

Communicating with patients and clients in ways that empower them to make informed choices about their health and healthcare and actively to promote their health and wellbeing

At novice level

Recognizing, having knowledge of and experiencing the role of a patient's advocate in communicating accurate information to patients in pain. Strategies used to empower them.

At intermediate level

Planning for, and application of, principles used in information giving, which include assessing the needs of the patient in pain, teaching others to use these skills and the psychosocial principles inherent in empowerment. Analysing the effectiveness of such principles and approaches.

Chapters 4, 5, 6, 8 and 9

Assessing individuals holistically, using a range of different assessment methods and reaching valid, reliable and comprehensive patient and client-centred conclusions that manage risk and are appropriate to needs, context and culture

At novice level

Recognizing the importance of, having knowledge of and experiencing responsibility for the care of a defined group of patients who may be in pain, using strategies to minimize risk, assessing patients' needs and recognizing own limitations as an accountable practitioner. Accessing available pain specialists for help and advice if they are required.

At intermediate level

Planning for, and applying, risk-management strategies and ensuring that the ward or team uses valid and reliable methods of pain and risk assessment. Educating the ward or team in assessment procedures and observing outcomes. Accepting and prioritizing pain-management referrals.

Chapters 6, 8, 9 and 10

Determining therapeutic programmes that are based on evidence, in the interests of patients and clients, and that involve other practitioners when this will improve health outcomes.

At novice level

Recognizing the importance of, having knowledge of, and being able to administer analgesic and therapeutic regimens as prescribed by other healthcare professionals following safe practice guidelines, supervision and training. Referring patients to available pain specialist nurses as patients' needs require.

At intermediate level

Planning for and applying therapeutic regimens safely, recommending analgesics from prescription protocols, and prescribing and administering nurse-led interventions in pain management. Educating the ward staff or team to manage patients in pain using evidence-based practice.

Chapters 6, 8, 9 and 10

Managing complete programmes of care effectively by working in partnership with others, delegating aspects to optimize health outcomes and resource use, and providing appropriate support to patients and clients.

At novice level

Recognizing, and having knowledge of and experience in providing support for the management of complete episodes of pain and care. Understanding the importance of holism in patient care and in pain management. Undertaking delegated care safely and in accordance with the wishes of the patient.

At intermediate level

Planning for and delegating aspects of total patient care to staff following assessment of patients' needs and staff abilities. Promoting holism in pain management and auditing care outcomes.

Chapters 1, 5, 7, 8 and 10

Making sound decisions, which are ethically based in the interests of patients and clients in the absence of precedents and protocols, in partnership with patients, clients and other professionals.

At novice level

Recognizing, and having knowledge and experience of, the basic ethical principles inherent in pain management and nursing. Understanding professional and legal responsibilities of the nurse in the care of patients. Seeking advice from senior colleagues when ethical problems arise, precedents do not exist and standard protocols do not apply. Supporting the patients in informed choice or in order to make ethical decisions.

At intermediate level

Responding to a lack of precedents and protocols by planning for and applying an ethical approach to assessing, managing and delegating care of patients in pain. Educating others in using legal and ethical principles. Supporting and helping the development of protocols and standards to address ethical issues. Appreciating ethnic diversity in developing strategies for ethical approaches to the management of pain in cultural groups.

References

Benner P (1984) From Novice to Expert. Sydney: Addison-Wesley.
The Pain Society (2002) Recommendations for Nursing Practice in Pain Management. London: The Pain Society.

Acknowledgements

We are indebted to all the contributors who gave their time and expertise to this book and for getting the chapters in on time. We would especially like to thank Audrey Clark for proofreading each chapter while using the principles of pacing to get through each without increasing her pain levels. We also thank all the patients who gave their time and encouragement while being interviewed for Chapter 3 (there are too many to list, but every one is special), and June Pears, a chronic pain sufferer, for providing such a heartfelt poem.

Introduction

It is often very difficult to manage chronic pain. Frequently there is no easy answer for the professional to give or for the patient to accept.

Chronic pain has different dimensions, which are often very much interwoven, so it is not always appropriate to use only one model of care. The medical model often refers to the organic causes of pain and needs to be involved in developing some of the answers. Patients with chronic diseases often develop chronic pain. However, not all patients suffering chronic pain can determine when or why the pain started.

This book will attempt to help the reader to understand the chronic pain experience from the perspective of the patient and the professional. It starts with an examination of models of care and works through the background of pain theories before looking at assessment and treatment strategies. The use of case presentations and learning objectives will challenge the reader to understand the links between the models and treatment/management strategies.

The authors acknowledge that it would be an impossible task to cover all options available for the treatment of chronic pain in this book. We feel that an understanding of acute pain has an important role to play in chronic pain, especially when acute pain is undertreated, so we have briefly discussed the link between acute and chronic episodes. We feel that it is important to explain some of the treatment strategies available to the professionals in developing planned episodes of care. Often the best way to manage a patient is by using multiple treatments. These treatments are not always developed sequentially – sometimes they overlap. We are also aware that many NHS trusts are unable to offer all that is available and presented within this book. Presenting them this way provides an opportunity for readers to challenge the merits of their practice as it stands now.

CHAPTER ONE

Models of health and illness

ANNIE SHELDRAKE

Aim

To provide an overview of the models used to understand chronic pain, the limitations inherent in the earlier models and the complexity needed to be incorporated in the later ones. To illustrate that the single most important factor in chronic pain management is that the individual is regarded as a whole, not a segment of compartmentalized pain.

Objectives

- To introduce the reader to a view that individuals with chronic pain need professionals and service provision that are focused on them as whole individual people rather than just body parts in pain.
- To provide an overview of models and theory construction in order that the reader can recognize different levels of explanation and how these impact upon understanding, care and treatment considerations.
- To provide the reader with an understanding of why the medical model is unsatisfactory when applied in isolation during the management of chronic pain.
- To highlight the development of thinking and model formulation with respect to chronic pain development and maintenance.
- To introduce the factors that are understood to contribute to a chronic pain experience and the models that have been formulated to meet current understanding.
- To provide a brief overview of a pain management programme.
- To illustrate the above with three case studies and draw together the presented points using the experiences of the three patients.

Chronic pain

It is impossible to imagine what it must be like to feel excruciating, unrelenting pain every waking moment of one's life – to have something so unavoidable impinge upon every conscious moment so that your very being becomes the pain and nothing else exists outside of it. Every attempt to make the pain go away fails, every explanation's inadequacy becomes apparent. Still the pain remains and along with it the belief, wish and hope that something or someone will make it all go away and that life can return to the way it was.

This is the domain of chronic pain. The overall prevalence of chronic pain found within the general population in a region of Scotland was 53.8% (Elliott et al., 2002). Shamefully, perhaps, in 2004 there was still no definitive explanation for its development or maintenance. Perhaps, however, this just highlights the complex issues and range of factors that seem to contribute to an experience of chronic pain. In the context of limited understanding it is easy to imagine why people – chronic pain sufferers and professionals alike – become frustrated, despondent and helpless. However, there is an increasing understanding of what chronic pain is not (curable) and a changing view, as a consequence, of how to realistically approach chronic pain management without being burdened by the unrealistic expectation of a cure.

In this chapter the changing perspective will be explored by examining the progress and use of conceptual models that have promoted and developed understanding. First, a brief overview of models and theory construction will be presented in order to establish recognition of their importance in directing conceptualization, care and treatment considerations. Secondly consideration will be given to the theory and models that have traditionally informed explanations of pain, examining the impact and limitations these have had with respect to understanding chronic pain.

These limitations can be seen to provide the forum from which current thinking has progressed. The factors that need to be considered in explanation of the development and maintenance of chronic pain will then be explored together with the way in which they have been encapsulated in the construction of current models and theory to understand chronic pain.

In particular, the need to consider chronic pain using a generic biopsychosocial model will be explored together with the way in which this has been incorporated, not only in the approach to assisting individuals but also as an essential component of chronic pain-management programmes (PMPs). Three cases will be presented to highlight the impact of different levels of explanation and intervention on the management of chronic pain.

Levels of explanation

Scientific enquiry is about seeking to understand observable phenomena. The enquiry embarks on a systematic process of gathering information that may be formulated to aid understanding and, in the case of clinical settings, used to improve direct care. Empirical generalization and theory formation are two levels of explanation at which scientific systematization occurs. The first relates directly to observable information including characteristics, events or attributes. The second, theory formation, refers to unobservable possible explanations of why the observable characteristics, events, attributes may go together. Different theoretical approaches will formulate different explanations. Theory formation is an important aspect of understanding as it develops from and generates testable hypotheses that, in turn, substantiate or repudiate the theoretical formulation.

A further conceptual level of scientific organization is that of models. Models are closely related to theories but are more accurate representations of reality, highlighting those elements of the world under investigation. For example, an engineer may study the effect of wind on a specific car shape by creating a model of the car shape. In social sciences a model is usually created with symbolic components and the relationships between them specified. Each type of model, both the physical and the symbolic, makes explicit the known relationships between each element of study.

Why is it important to consider levels of explanation with respect to understanding chronic pain? A simplistic answer is that chronic pain is still viewed from a largely monocular, if dichotomous, perceptive. Traditionally a physical cause needed to be established, with the assumption that this could be eliminated or anaesthetized. If no physical cause was established the pain was labelled 'idiopathic'. It was then attributed to psychological causes with the implication that pain exists 'in people's minds'. By implication, the pain is then regarded by medical professionals as not real and the individual is seen as 'making it up'. Chronic pain, then, was regarded as either organic or psychological. Almost without exception, those suffering chronic pain have been on the receiving end of this belief system. Not only does this end up ensuring that they feel helpless and alone, it does not bring understanding of chronic pain any closer as these two positions are clearly inadequate explanations when considered in such a mutually exclusive way.

The less simplistic answer is that chronic pain develops over time and persists long after a physiological cause is assumed to have ceased. This persistence, in the absence of physiological factors, is curious and has challenged assumptions that pain is experienced only in the presence of noxious stimuli. Essentially pain can become benign but intractable.

The perception of pain therefore does not appear to 'behave' in a linear manner, remaining long after the original injury has receded and healed. As a consequence the management of chronic pain has challenged both medical and psychological understanding, remaining a particularly difficult problem.

The medical model

In medicine the medical model is perhaps the most familiar and prominent example of a symbolic representation of reality. The medical model in essence reflects an understanding about pathological processes by identifying observable consistent patterns of symptoms, their causes and the course of these symptoms. This model is primarily a disease model reflecting organic processes and does not include the role of psychological or social factors. It is a persuasive and powerful model that has, as a result, generated a fantastical faith in its ability to restore and cure.

Although the medical model is really a very pure linear model it is often used very generally when describing processes that appear to involve physical states to be managed by physiological means. In fact Bonica (1990) suggests that in chronic pain it is the pain that is the disease as it has become the malevolent force.

On the face of it, pain does appear to reside in the field of medicine, occurring as it does in the physical body. As a consequence the tools available to medicine – medication, surgery and physiotherapy – are, where necessary, applied to the management of the pain. The problem is that when pain becomes chronic it does not seem to respond at all well to these tools. In fact in many cases these tools may compound the problem and create different problems including doctor shopping, excessive pharmacological intervention, intrusive surgery, and increasing disability and suffering. It could be argued that this also reflects a poor understanding by physicians both of the state of being human and of the somewhat distorted use of the medical model. The fact is that the effects of environmental social events, psychological factors and emotions are all translated, interpreted and responded to by neurophysiological systems. These neurophysiological systems are sophisticated, holistic representations of us that do not exclude our perceptions and interpretations of our world and can exert precision conditioning and reconditioning. They are quite capable of distorting pain perception, increasing disability, and producing severe and unrelenting nociception. However, the medical model framework tends to be used without due respect to this level of neurophysiological sophistication and, as applied to chronic pain management, largely continues to exclude and ignore the multiple other factors that are implicated in chronic pain development.

As stated, pain has traditionally (and still is to a large extent) been considered from the perspective of a medical model. As the setting for most management of pain is in a hospital by medical-model-trained staff the questions for attention are primarily diagnostic and relate to cure. Which medical practitioner examines the pain will depend largely on which part of the body the pain occurs in and consideration is generally centred on the area of the body the pain manifests in. This is reinforced by the fact that most individuals know exactly where they are feeling the physical pain and generally have an exact knowledge when they acquired it.

During our pain-management programme, the pain anaesthetist used a wonderful analogy to help people understand this process. Imagine an elephant. Each specialist doctor has a particular part of the elephant that they are considering. If the medic is a tail specialist he or she is unlikely to consider the trunk. If the medic is an ear specialist he or she is unlikely to consider the stomach. And so forth. In fact they might not even recognize that they are dealing with a whole fully functioning elephant (it is a long way from one end of an elephant to the other!). This selective view of the elephant is important as it informs and increases understanding of specific parts, which are often very complex and specialized. However, the danger is that by not considering the whole elephant the view may be too selective and miss other things that are contributing to the problem. For sake of imagination, it may be that the poor elephant's trunk is sore because he is not eating the correct diet (organic/environmental), that he is bored and is using his trunk to ease his boredom (psychological) and that his trunk has become the object of another elephant's attention because it is also bored (social/environmental).

In response to their specific areas of expertise the experts also have a bag of specific and highly specialized medical interventions that they can use to 'treat' the part they are experts in. Added to this is the complication that the elephant really does want to feel well again so he will try anything. This is a jointly experienced pressure between the specialist and the elephant (psychosocial).

In most medical situations this compartmentalizing is acceptable and necessary and does not, in fact, create problems. However, in some areas of medicine, such as rehabilitation, palliative care, oncology and chronic pain, this view is considered to be too selective and does not provide a breadth of understanding about the individual to improve functioning. It could be argued that the aim of all interventions is to achieve functional restoration and this often necessitates consideration of the individual's psychological and social world as well as their physical one.

Early explanations of pain reflected this linear compartmentalized view. These included 'specificity' theory proposed by Muller in 1842 and 'pattern' theory proposed by Goldscheider in 1894 (for a comprehensive overview see

Melzack and Wall, 1996). Both perspectives considered pain purely as a physiological sensory response. However, these sensory models of pain were limited in predicative abilities and unable to explain a number of observable and interesting phenomena, which present as puzzling if nothing else.

The example of Beecher's (1956) account of soldiers, wounded at Anzio, is consistently quoted as highlighting the complex issue of pain itself. Soldiers returned with penetrating and horrendous injuries, required no analgesics and reported that they were not in significant pain. This, and laboratory work, led Beecher (1960) to draw a conclusion that no simple relationship exists between a stimulus that elicits pain and a response. At the other extreme is the butcher who, while hanging meat, suspended himself by the hook. Terrified he cried out in excessive pain. The hook, however, had not touched his arm – it had merely pierced his coat (Tuke, 1884). Both of these examples implicate the influence of meaning on the experience of pain, anticipation of future consequences and memory.

Other observations that theoretical understanding needs to explain include:

- amputees who are often in extreme and continual pain long after their wound and limb have been removed;
- pain often spreads from the site of the original injury to unpredicted and unrelated areas of the body;
- pain can persist even after the connections between the peripheral and central nervous systems have been surgically severed;
- pain can be reactivated by the gentlest stimuli and occur without the presence of any apparent stimulus;
- pain can become chronic and intractable.

Psychological explanations

Labelling chronic pain as 'idiopathic' led to a whole new area of explanation involving psychological exploration of individual characteristics that might have been causing the pain. Psychodynamic theorists regarded intractable pain as an expression of emotional disturbance arising from unconscious and unresolved conflicts. Conceptualizing chronic pain in this way led to research that examined the aetiological significance of early family relationships, socio-economic status, birth order, marital adjustment, depression and personality disorders. However, aetiological evidence is largely unsubstantiated and of questionable significance (Roy, 1985; Gamsa, 1990). Gamsa (1994) summarizes that, whereas there may be some individuals whose pain is caused by emotional conflict, a purely psychological explanation is not satisfactory for most people and again fails to consider the complexity of the presenting issues.

Behaviourists such as Fordyce et al. (1968) believed that the development of pain into a chronic state, and the maintenance of this state, occurs because pain behaviours such as facial and postural expression, verbalization, medication use and seeking medical explanation become reinforced. Taking the view that it is only through these behaviours that any of us can know that someone is in pain they proposed that these behaviours occur for two reasons: first as a 'respondent', which is the nociceptive (a nociceptor is a receptor preferentially sensitive to noxious stimuli) reflex to stimulation; second, as an operant, sensitive to pain-reinforcing consequences. Chronic pain, it is suggested, is the consequence of pain behaviours being reinforced long after the respondent element of the original injury has ceased. As a consequence a behavioural treatment for chronic pain would be to eliminate contingent behaviours (Turks and Rudy, 1983; Fordyce, Roberts and Sternback, 1985) and replace them with 'well behaviours'. A decrease in pain behaviour is therefore identified as treatment success.

That pain behaviours can be demonstrated to be under control of environmental influences does indicate that they may become maladaptive patterns of behaviour and open to amelioration. However, to regard pain behaviours as the sole contributor to chronic pain after the noxious stimuli are no longer present is also a linear perspective about the experience of pain. More importantly, though, just because people do not *show* that they are in pain does not mean they *are* not in pain. Often individuals in chronic pain will go to great lengths to 'hide' their suffering from family and friends, especially when they have been in pain for many years. This in itself can present as a problem, undermining the intimate levels of a relationship.

Investigation by cognitive theorists on intervening variables such as expectations, self-statements, beliefs, self-efficacy, attributions, locus of control and coping styles have established that these factors also contribute to the experience of pain (Turk and Rudy, 1983; Bandura et al., 1987; Turner 1991). Cognitive interventions that challenge meanings and thought patterns have been found to be effective in reducing the experience of pain and improving quality of life (Herman and Bapiste, 1981; Nicholas, Wilson and Goyen, 1992). These aspects will be considered where relevant later in the chapter and relate to a cognitive–behavioural understanding often incorporated in PMPs.

Biopsychosocial explanation

This is not a precision model but its tenet is central to understanding present conceptualizations of chronic pain. This is that there are three areas of interactive influence that affect an individual:

1. the *physiological* state of the individual's body, organs and organic processes;

2. the individual's *psychological* world, including interpretations, thoughts, feelings, responses (both internal and external) and learning; and
3. the individual's *external social/environmental* world. This includes the family such individuals live with, the family they were brought up by, the cultural context they live in, and the type and sources of information to which they respond.

These three areas are assumed to be intimately related and influential on each other. In using such a model there needs to be consideration and exploration of how, what, where and why each area contributes to the presenting observable phenomenon.

The evidence for considering chronic pain from the perspective of a biopsychosocial model is that the pain will not have eased with recovery, will probably have increased in sensitivity, lowering thresholds and increasing intensity, and will probably be poorly controlled by traditional methods. Poor control leads to psychological trauma, increasing emotional distress and creating a whole range of secondary debilitating problems. These include increased levels of anxiety and depression, fear of disability and societal stigmatization. Anger, frustration, helplessness, hopelessness and inadequacy are all commonly reported feelings associated with being in chronic pain. A significant decrease in all activities occurs and life is less likely to be seen as pleasurable. Increasing isolation and changes in intimate relationships are common. Socio-economic status often changes, which can cause further distress and suffering.

Case example: AD

To highlight the multiple levels of influence and the journey that an individual might take let us consider AD – a 57-year-old man who, in 1993, lifted a weight that he estimated as being twice as heavy as a 56 lb bag of potatoes. After a few days of intense pain he went to his GP who recommended seeing an osteopath. This proved unhelpful as the osteopath suspected he had a prolapsed disc. Eventually, after a number of weeks of physiotherapy to gain some mobility, he was admitted for surgery to have his L4–5 and L5–S1 discs removed. Decompression surgery was necessary again a few weeks later at L2 – the sacrum. For a few days after each surgical intervention AD was pain free. However, within days the pain had returned. AD describes these initial months as the 'start of a long road of despair, as I could not accept what had gone wrong'.

AD then embarked on a process of trying to find pain relief. He received monthly epidurals, midazolam spinal injections and finally, in 1998, a spinal-cord stimulator was implanted following comprehensive physical and psychological assessment. At the same time as receiving all these he was being prescribed a range of pharmaceutical interventions among which were amitriptyline, morphine sulphate, carbamazepine and tramadol. (See Chapter 6 for discussion on interventions and Chapter 9 for medication.) At the time of our first meeting he reported taking three non-steroidal anti-inflammatory drugs (NSAIDs), slow-release morphine, an antidepressant and an anticonvulsant.

> The funny part about it [was] none of it was really giving much pain relief. I was getting more and more depressed. I think my family felt it more than I did as I was really not in control. After two years of all this medication I was a zombie in a lot of pain.

It is helpful here to consider who this man is. AD presents as an extremely self-reliant man who likes to feel that he is in total control. He can be cantankerous, single-minded, sceptical and suspicious. He holds fixed beliefs about things and has a strong sense of duty and traditional role values. He is determined and courageous as well as fragile and vulnerable. He requires straight answers to straight questions and does 'not suffer fools'. In 1964 he fell 38 feet, suffered a crush fracture and walked 7 miles to the nearest hospital because he did not want to 'bother anyone'. He discharged himself from hospital when they recommended 2 weeks' traction – because he was getting married. In essence AD's life was determined by his perception of being in control and being able to manage anything and everything. However, the experiences following his injury in 1993 began a process of challenge and change for AD.

> I felt so useless as a man having been so independent all my life and never asking anyone to do anything for me. I now had to ask for help with just about everything and that was so degrading. I felt when my wife was carrying the heavy bags and I nothing, that people were saying, 'look at that big bloke letting his little wife carry those bags'. Over a period of time this slowly built up without me realizing what was going on.

This poignant comment by AD highlights the need for a multifactorial biopsychosocial model, to help unpack all the influences associated with the pain and AD's and others' responses to it. The suffering individual's experience cannot be stressed enough. AD had experienced a physical injury with a severity that very quickly needed surgical intervention. It may have removed the cause – the prolapsed discs – but he continued to be in severe, debilitating pain. This pain drove him to take increasingly large amounts of medication, including morphine, and endure significant intrusive medical interventions. Over time this impacted significantly on his mood and his ability to live his life independently. Initially AD attributes much of this to the tablets he was taking. However, psychologically he was increasingly struggling with many changes and losses. His role as a man and all the levels of responsibility he attributed to the role had changed and he was no longer able to identify himself in society or with his family as a valuable member. His sense of self-worth was decreasing and as a consequence he was increasingly feeling inadequate and suicidal. At this stage AD was referred to the pain-management programme for assessment (discussed later).

The biopsychosocial model provides an important perspective on chronic pain. As Gallager (1999: 825) points out 'not only does chronic pain not have an anatomic and neurophysiologic substrate, but also involves the conditioning of the neurophysiologic systems both by the pain itself and by psychosocial experience'. The effective treatment of chronic pain demands, then, that individuals are considered from a multidimensional perspective that includes consideration of their physical, psychological and social states.

One of the important and significant uses of the biopsychosocial model should be in its application in clinical practice prior to the pain reaching a chronic state – less than 12 weeks. Failure to consider a prolonged experience of pain from a multidimensional perspective is likely to lead into a well-documented process of doctor shopping, high medication use, decreased psychological control and coping, increasing use of intrusive interventions, and an inevitable and predictable decline in psychological and social wellbeing. Gallagher argues that using the biopsychosocial model enables the clinician to take an analytic approach. This is then used to elucidate the relevant information, organize it categorically and reach a workable formulation/hypothesis. This formulation directs coordinated treatment, ensures early referral to specialist pain-management professionals, and identifies priority problem areas and subsequent goal management. The model therefore provides a systematic and conceptual means of considering the complexity of chronic pain, its development, maintenance and points at which intervention may be most effective.

One impact of using a biopsychosocial approach early on is that it acts as a systematic guide for all clinicians involved. This increases understanding of what is and is not achievable. It helps move the clinician from a position of trying to cure to one of achieving pain control and preventing functional deterioration. This increases the opportunity to develop more realistic goals and limit the indiscriminate use of medication and intrusive surgical interventions. In neurophysiological terms there is also the opportunity to prevent any permanent damage/change to finely balanced neurophysiological systems. Familiarity and adoption of the biopsychosocial model at all levels in healthcare, from primary care through to secondary care, ensures that the individual is at all times represented holistically in the mind of the clinician.

A second impact of using the model is for individuals and their families, enabling them to gain an understanding of the potential relationships between the contributing factors. The reasons why individuals seek advice, from whom they seek it, and what they then do with the advice when they are unwell, are complex and by no means fully understood (for a comprehensive and interesting review see Skevington, 1995). However, most people (Weiner, 1985) actively seek a causal explanation. The question 'why?' is felt by Weiner to occur when an individual is facing a situation of great importance where loss, stress or unexpected outcomes are involved. The attributions that they use to explain the causes have been found to link closely with an individual's perception of responsibility and control (Rotter, 1966). During a biopsychosocial consultation the clinician is more rapidly able to establish an understanding of these factors. This can then be used to assist individuals to consider their causal explanations, attributions and the degree of personal responsibility they take for managing the pain. The consultation process itself acts as an intervention opportunity as the individual is encouraged to consider a multidimensional understanding of their pain. This can begin a process of empowerment to take back control rather than relinquishing it to the pain, the physician or the medication.

Providing an opportunity to consider their ongoing pain as a complex interrelationship is an educational process and one that is fundamental. The biopsychosocial model provides an important conceptual model to assist in this education process. Education improves understanding, dispels myths, reduces helpless feelings, enables individuals to learn about themselves and their bodies, and provides them with an important rationale for the treatment interventions they are being encouraged to use such as relaxation, exercise and pacing.

The model is an important means to conceptualize an understanding of the complexity of issues that appear to contribute to the development and maintenance of pain into a chronic state. It enables a wide range of perspectives to be considered and can help to prevent some of the inherent difficulties associated with a linear model. The biopsychosocial model is an integrated umbrella model that subsumes a variety of different theories and models from each of the three areas. These include the gate-control theory and the cognitive–behavioural model.

The gate-control theory

The biopsychosocial model provides a generic conceptualization of the areas of influence in chronic pain but it is the gate-control theory that has drawn together research and phenomenological information and conceptualized the physiological structures to account for many of the above observations.

Conceptualized by Melzack and Wall in 1965, it is the most influential and current working physiological model of pain. This theory is not entirely satisfactory in that aspects of it remain hypothetical and assumptions are made about the properties of the nervous system including the neural pathways and structures involved. However the essential strength of the model is the identification of top-down processes such as inhibitory descending pathways and the identification of brain structures related to learning and avoidance of pain through pain memories. These are understood to have a significant influence in the modulation of pain and relate to psychological factors.

In summary, the theory proposes that stimulation is detected by fast, large afferents and slow, small afferents terminating in the substantia gelatinosa (SG) of the dorsal horn of the spinal column. Impulses from these afferents are 'summed' in the SG. Impulses are then transmitted to the central transmission cells or T cells, also situated in the dorsal horn of the spinal cord. Output to the T cells depends on the summing process in the SG. Activation by a large, fast fibre will excite the suppressor cells, closing the gate. Small, slow fibres open the gate by inhibiting the suppressor cells that activate the T cells. The balance between the inhibitory and excitatory impulses is critical to the firing of the T cells. If large, fast fibres are reduced in number as a consequence of damage then impulses from the small, slow fibres are excessive, the gate remains open and pain continues. T cell output transmits information to the local reflex circuits and the brain.

Pain is identified and evaluated by the brain in terms of its physical properties and past experience. This evaluation activates cognitive, affective and motivational systems in the frontal cortex. Connections with the frontal cortex and the structures in the limbic system account for the strong interplay between emotion and higher order evaluation. The theory also proposes that escape from and avoidance of pain are learned. Centres in the intralaminar and medial nuclei of the thalamus match incoming information with memories of past experiences, enabling learning to take place and be consolidated (Wall and Melzack, 1983).

The gate-control theory has the potential to incorporate observed patterns of pain and acknowledges the probable role of higher cortical processes. Melzack's (1973) view is that pain has three components: sensory–discriminative, motivational–affective and cognitive–evaluative. The identification of higher-level integration in the experience of pain is important as it implicates the role of psychological and social elements as well.

The cognitive–behavioural model

In the early 1960s and 1970s, behavioural management was used to treat chronic pain (see review Fordyce, 1968, 1973). This is significant as behavioural management is based on learning theory. Learning theory identified and developed by researchers such as Ivan Pavlov (1849–1936) and Edward Thorndike (1874–1949) is extremely important to our understanding of both animal and human behaviour. Learning theory postulates a number of important things about how we learn to behave in the way we do. Behaviour is anything that we can observe/see both in others and in ourselves. Moving your hand to scratch your head is a behaviour as is watching somebody grimace and hold their back as they get up. Behaviours are happening all the time in every situation where people or animals are.

In brief, learning occurs because there are consequences of behaving in a particular way. How we behave affects how others behave to us and how others behave affects how we behave to them.

This is called the ABC of behaviour. It stands for:

- Antecedent – the circumstances or situation prior to the behaviour;
- Behaviour – how we respond to the antecedent/consequence;
- Consequence – the effect that that behaviour has on subsequent behaviours that will follow from it.

This is an intricate ongoing process where one behaviour becomes the consequence and antecedent for another and so on ad infinitum.

Behaviours are learned in this process through three primary routes:

- By *association or classical conditioning*. If we're hungry we eat; if we are thirsty we drink. If we burn ourselves on a flame we remove ourselves from harm.
- Through *reinforcement or operant learning*. Things or events that we enjoy and things that we avoid because we don't enjoy them are called operants or reinforcers. An operant can be anything that increases the likelihood of the behaviour being repeated. Operants may be helpful or unhelpful in terms of chronic pain but they will always lead to an increase in a particular behaviour. So if people find that the pain is less if they don't do anything, they will stop doing things and thereby avoid the pain (avoidance learning) and increase the probability of not doing things in the future. In a similar manner if we have a headache we take pain-relieving medication because we have learned that it leads to a reduction in the pain. Demonstrated in AD's observation, however, is one of the problems associated with such solid learning: pain medication continues to be taken long after it has stopped working in the way we have learned.
- We also learn not do things through *punishment*. Punishment is any aversive stimulus that occurs following an operant behaviour and decreases the likelihood of that behaviour being produced again.

Through association, reinforcement and punishment, patterns of behaviour are learned and unlearned and new ones learned to replace them. Set patterns of behaviour develop between people and by people. These patterns may or may not always be helpful for us as individuals but they can be difficult to change because each behaviour is part of an ABC responding process.

In the context of pain it is true to say that we know that people are in pain only if they tell us and/or they behave in a way that leads us, as observers, to infer that they are in pain. Without pain behaviour we would not know. There are multitudes of pain behaviours including facial expression, medication use, verbal tone, posture and inactivity. All of these behaviours are subject to the same routes of learning and development of behaviour patterns both by the individual in pain and by the people who respond to them. The role of avoidance learning, contingent reinforcers, conditioned aversive stimuli and the lack of well behaviours have all been identified as significant in the development of chronic pain behaviours, as has the role of significant others and health professionals who are considered important in contingency learning associated with pain behaviours.

In a typical behavioural PMP, pain behaviours are identified and then ignored (Cairns, 1976). One aims to reduce or eliminate medication, a contingent behaviour, and family members are provided with information about reinforcement and the importance of ignoring pain behaviours. Activity levels are increased to counteract physical de-conditioning and goals established for effective reinforcement of well behaviours (Fordyce et al., 1968; Fordyce 1976).

Authors such as Roberts and Reinhardt (1980) concluded from running behavioural groups that a significant amount of chronic disability in people with chronic pain is due to learned behaviour and that behavioural programmes prevented and reduced chronic pain and associated disability through the reduction of reinforcements of pain behaviours.

However, programmes that these authors and others ran were criticized for neglecting the myriad of other factors that could have been contributing to improvement, that levels of stoicism were increased rather than the pain being treated (Schmidt, 1987) and that they failed to meet individual needs (Merskey, 1985). Although these are valid criticisms, the roles of pain behaviours and learning are important factors to consider in formulating a biopsychosocial understanding of a person's response to pain.

Pure behavioural approaches to pain management are no longer considered appropriate but attention is always drawn to the role of pain behaviours when considering factors associated with chronic pain management. Put simply, if someone is 'gaining' from their pain continuing then these behaviours need to be considered as a possible contributing element. This whole question regarding the function of the pain for the individual is probably highlighted most when litigation issues are pending. As a clinician it is also one of the hardest aspects to approach with some people. It needs to be done in a timely manner and when trust and engagement have been established.

As a personal observation, it appears that people gain from their pain because they are unable to find more appropriate means of having their needs met. In one PMP a young mother with a large family and a multitude of financial worries discovered that she 'used' her pain to create space for herself. It gave her permission to leave her duties and spend time alone. Work with her focused on finding more appropriate strategies to manage and cope with the demands placed on her and on identifying specific 'her time'. As a consequence her pain became less prominent and problematic.

As a consequence of the limitations associated with behavioural programmes and evidence of the role of cognitive factors in chronic pain treatment a more general cognitive–behavioural approach (Skinner et al., 1990) is used to help formulate a psychological understanding of a person's responses to pain.

The cognitive–behavioural model is an important conceptual model used for considering the impact, development and management of chronic pain. This model was first proposed by Aaron Beck (1976) as a cognitive therapy model for the treatment of emotional disorders. Beck approached emotional disorders from the perspective that 'Man has the key to understanding and solving his psychological disturbance within the scope of his own awareness' (Beck, 1976: 3). This is achieved through correcting misconceptions and problem solving using thought and thinking as a consciously available source of information. Beck argues that an individual, through observation and consideration of his or her thoughts, wishes, feelings and actions, is capable of self-monitoring and self-instruction. By becoming aware of these thinking patterns – specifically those that are unhelpful and destructive – individuals can begin to challenge and restate their position in a more helpful and productive manner.

Cognitive–behavioural treatments have grown in popularity and have developed from Beck's original thinking. The model is an integral part of all mental health services and is increasingly being employed in many areas of health psychology. In considering chronic pain the premise is that idiosyncratic attitudes, beliefs, attributions, expectations, memories and assumptions interact with sensory, behavioural and emotional factors. Thought patterns, feeling states and coping skills exert an important influence on nociception, on the level of distress and suffering experienced, and on individual disability and adjustment.

Individuals are introduced to the concept that there is an intimate interaction and influence exerted by five areas of life experience (Greenberger and Padesky, 1995 – see Figure 1.1). These five areas are thinking, feeling, behaviour, physical responses and the environment (the biopsychosocial model):

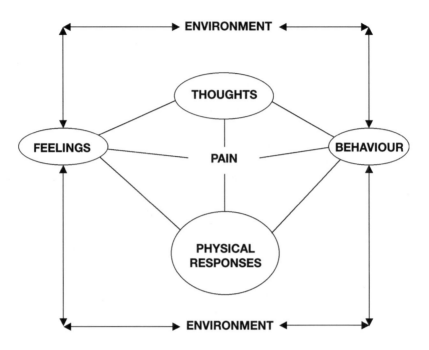

Figure 1.1 Model of influencing interactions.

- *Thinking.* This refers to the aspect of us that arguably makes us human. Thoughts are constant and continual even if we are not always conscious of them. They are not observable and they are generally automatic – they just pop into our heads.
- *Feelings.* These are a reflection of our emotional world and experiences. They are also constant and continual. We may not always be consciously aware of them and they are also unobservable to others. However, we recognize them in others through behaviour and one-word labels such as anger, sadness, happiness. Feelings have different intensities and sometimes it is possible to muddle feelings up – for example, by thinking that we are feeling anger when we are feeling anxious. This may occur because our physical autonomic response to both these feeling states is very, very similar. We may also experience several feelings at once.
- *Behaviour.* This is any response, act or activity. Behaviours are always observable by others. They are constant and continuous. We are constantly but unconsciously revising behavioural patterns as a consequence of learning from changing environmental demands. Behaviours can be difficult to label accurately given that they are also directed by people's internal unobservable world of thoughts and feelings.

- *Physical reactions.* These are any and all of the body's responses to both internal and external stimuli. They include such things as heart rate, dizziness, shaking, muscle tension, sweating, breathing, 'butterflies', headaches, pain and so forth.
- *Environment.* This is anything external to individuals both from their past and in their present. Environmental influences include family, culture, gender, neighbours, religion and media. It also includes learned beliefs and expectations that we have about our environment as these have been formed by the aspects of our environment. In essence we do not exist in a bubble isolated from the impact of the world around us and the world around us can have a profound impact on our internal world (thoughts and feelings) and behaviour.

These five areas are considered to affect the experience of pain both in a helpful way by decreasing the experience of pain and in an unhelpful way by increasing the experience of pain depending on the influence of each area at the time.

For example, individuals may think that their pain will never be less than it is. This may lead to their feeling increasingly despondent, frustrated, miserable and sorry for themselves. Behaviour is likely to reflect these feelings. As activity reduces, physical deconditioning occurs, which increases the likelihood of pain persisting (in evolutionary terms our physical health ensures our survival). From each of these interconnections the experience of pain can be increased, decreasing self-worth and increasing unhelpful thought patterns and behaviour.

If, however, individuals think that, although their pain is bad today, if they relax and do something pleasant, then in a few minutes or hours it will be less painful, they can move onto something else. They are more likely to experience feelings of control rather than helplessness and helpful thoughts rather than bleak, unhelpful thoughts. Consider for a moment a thought that you last had about yourself and the impact this had upon how you felt, what you then did and the impact on your next set of thoughts.

By shifting thinking in this way, and learning how these five areas relate to and influence each other, individuals are able to begin considering themselves and their pain in a different light. They can move from being people in *pain* to *people* in pain.

It is the latter position that many people have lost as the pain has invaded every aspect of their life and consciousness. They have often lost their sense of themselves and the things they need and enjoy as a person relinquishing these things in a misguided attempt to try to control the pain. As AD's comments highlight, this is often an insidious and gradual process that takes over the person. Assisting people to consider the above interactions is not easy but most people (not all) are able to begin to identify changes in their pain experience as they learn how their whole beings interact and impact upon it. It is also of course a model of living as well and many people benefit from the opportunity to reflect and think upon the powerful impact of these influences in all aspects of their lives.

Summary

The amount of research on pain and chronic pain has generally been determined by individual theoretical positions. This effectively led to singular treatment approaches such as medication, behavioural programmes and family therapy.

Adopting a multifactorial approach has increasingly been the challenge for a modern working conceptualization of chronic pain. Greater understanding regarding the potential role of a variety of factors (physical, behavioural, cognitive and social) in the development and maintenance of chronic pain indicates this, as have the ongoing limitations with traditional treatments. Clearer scientific understanding and the development of the gate-control theory, which incorporates understanding of the ascending and descending central nervous system, has provided a schematic representation of how these factors impact upon pain perception.

Pain management

Increasing scientific exploration and explanation, leading to the evolution of the biopsychosocial model as the best representation of how to approach the problems associated with chronic pain, suggested a need for a multidisciplinary approach to the management and treatment of chronic pain. In 1960, Dr J Bonica, an American anaesthesiologist, recognized that there was no single specialist who could manage the complexity of difficulties presented by people in chronic pain. The need for a multidisciplinary approach was therefore identified. This provides the most appropriate means of using the model and ensures individual professional disciplines involvement. The development of PMPs was a next step in this progress. These are structured programmes currently endorsed by the Association of Anaesthetists of Great Britain and Northern Ireland and the Pain Society.

General aims of pain-management programmes

The aim of PMPs as stated by the Pain Society (1997) 'is to reduce the disability and distress caused by chronic pain by teaching sufferers physical, psychological and practical techniques to improve their quality of life. It differs from other treatment provided in pain clinics in that pain relief is not the primary goal'.

Hendler (1981) regards the aim of PMPs as a process of rehabilitation that fosters self-reliance. The aims adopted by PMPs are not about delivering a pain-free existence or a cure. In adopting this particular position sufferers and professionals are removed from these constricting and unrealistic expectations (Eccelston, Williams and Stainton, 1997).

Structure and content

Pain-management programmes assume a number of things that inform the structure and content:

- that pain is not consistent over time;
- that the experience of pain is complicated;
- that pain is multifaceted;
- that not enough is known about pain to 'promise' no pain; and
- that people can be helped to gain a greater degree of control over the pain experience through education and taught techniques.

Pain-management programmes treat groups of individuals as inpatients or as outpatients. Gentry and Owen (1986) identify seven clinical reasons for group work with chronic pain sufferers. These include, for clients, the common problems they face, economical use of time, amelioration of social isolation factors, credible feedback, alternative perspectives, a new reference group and for the therapist the reduced chance of dependency.

The structure and content of PMPs fit broadly into the categories of education, group discussion and skills training. Of interest is a comment by Weir, Woodside and Crook (1988) on PMPs. They suggest that 'difficulties in understanding, describing and teaching the treatment process [of the PMP are] that several different conceptual models are implicitly used in the clinical formulation and subsequent therapeutic approaches but rarely identified as such' (Weir et al., 1988: 109).

As stated above, the two models generally associated with directing the content of PMPs are the cognitive–behavioural model and the gate-control theory. Pain-management programmes typically introduce the gate-control theory as this provides an opportunity for clinicians to introduce the role of higher descending cortical influences and to challenge beliefs about pain as more than an organic response. Turk and Rudy (1983) refer to this as 're-conceptualizing the problem'. It also provides an opportunity for individuals to recognize that they can close pain gates and, by doing so, decrease the pain threshold.

Beliefs about pain and its causes are regarded as an important challenge for PMPs. Edwards et al. (1992) compared the beliefs of people in pain and people not in pain. Individuals not in pain believed that psychological factors such as thought patterns, coping and anxiety could all influence pain. Individuals in pain regarded their pain as organic and tended to deny psychological influences. Jensen, Karoly and Huger (1987) identified five beliefs held by chronic pain sufferers:

1. that a doctor will get rid of the pain;
2. that they are not in control of the pain;
3. that others are responsible for helping when a person is in pain;
4. that pain is permanent and leads to disability and an inability to work;
5. that medication is the most useful.

These beliefs tend to highlight the reason why PMPs aim to develop self-reliance and a sense of greater personal control.

Skills training

Increasing perceived control is central to the task of PMPs and therefore skills training through practice and education is at the heart of the programmes. A number of different skills are incorporated including relaxation, increasing exercise and activity levels, pacing, challenging pain behaviours and unhelpful thinking patterns, and developing strategies for coping.

Relaxation

A significant emphasis in PMPs is on teaching skills such as decreasing levels of muscle tension and lowering autonomic arousal. This increases an individual's awareness of their physical responses to the pain and other influences. Tension and relaxation are mutually exclusive states and therefore cannot occur at the same time. However, studies that have assessed whether there is a link between pain and physical changes such as muscle tension, vascular changes and autonomic arousal are extensive but generally inconclusive. Flor and Turk (1989) reviewed 47 studies that considered the relationship between these physiological responses and pain in people with tension headaches, lower back pain and temporomandibular pain. They found no evidence of an elevated or different physiology. They did, however, identify that stressful events are linked to physiological changes. This is significant because pain is generally regarded as a stressor.

A number of studies investigated the benefits of relaxation or biofeedback based on the rationale that pain is a stressor. Evidence collected

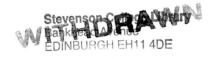

indicates that biofeedback and relaxation can alleviate pain (Haynes et al., 1975; Blanchard et al., 1978; Keefe et al., 1981; Linton, 1984). Cox, Freundlich and Meyer (1975) compared biofeedback, relaxation and medication placebo in 27 individuals with chronic tension headaches. Relaxation and biofeedback were equally as effective, but were superior to medicine placebo post-assessment and at 4-month follow-up. Linton and Gotestarn (1984) demonstrated that relaxation was just as effective as behavioural programmes. However, there may be differential effects with behavioural programmes – for example, reducing medication use and increasing activity.

A review by Turner and Chapman (1982) concluded that although these methods are used in PMPs there is little direct evidence to support the assumptions on which they are practised, namely that they reduce muscle tension and lower arousal. Furthermore the reasons why these treatments are effective are poorly understood but it may be that they provide an extra resource and/or increase an individual's perception of control and coping.

Exercise and activity

Lack of exercise and poor fitness have been associated with above-normal levels of negative emotions, anxiety, confusion, anger, tension and depression (Sheehan, 1994) and exercise is regarded as a significant contributor to health and wellbeing. Exercise and improving fitness play a central role in PMPs. Physical deconditioning leads to poor muscle strength, flexibility, endurance and low mood. Individuals generally believe that they will do even more damage if they exercise. They may feel frightened when they start exercising after a period of inactivity because they hurt. However, this is a normal physical response. It highlights the interaction of thoughts, feelings, behaviour and physical response in decreasing activity.

Pacing

Individuals in pain tend to be active when their pain feels less. During these periods of activity the tendency is to do as much as they can and to excess. This often causes several days of severe discomfort. It develops into an unhelpful pattern, which eventually reduces activity levels to virtually nothing.

Pacing is a technique that involves doing less more often and planning equal levels of activity each day. The associated loss of physical fitness as exercise decreases, excessive discomfort following periods of activity, avoidance behaviours and an increase in unhelpful thinking and emotions support the inclusion of exercise in PMPs (see Chapter 8).

Stress and coping

Banks and Kerns (1996) identified pain as a particularly potent and unique stressor. They conclude that pain is nearly always aversive and has the ability to pervade consciousness in a manner that is all too often inescapable. This is partly supported by 35% of volunteers who identified their lower back pain as the most stressful aspect in their lives. However, it is not clear how many other stresses individuals had in their life generally.

Pain is also stressful in that cognitive appraisal of it may determine that the pain is dangerous. In acute pain this is often the case and it is a timely warning to stop. However, attributing chronic pain to danger arouses anxiety, particularly when the pain persists after self-medication and medical interventions have been tried. Anxiety becomes a fear of lasting pain, that the pain will be progressive and associated with disability, and that the pain signals an underlying disease. Constant and inescapable anxiety leads to high levels of stress as individuals find themselves in a position that they are unable to influence.

The symptoms of this associated anxiety can include somatic, cognitive, intense feelings and escape avoidance behaviours (Lethern et al., 1983; Fernandez and Turk, 1992; LaRocca, 1992; McCraken, Zayfert and Gross, 1992). Sequelae of chronic pain, such as loss of job, relationship difficulties and disability, are also significant stressors. These and the associated fears contribute to the stress of pain so that individuals may often be at their limit in terms of implementing cognitive and behavioural coping strategies and tolerating the emotionality of pain (Banks and Kerns, 1996).

Cognitive models such as stress inoculation training (Meichenbaum, 1977) have had an important influence on current PMPs, specifically because the training emphasizes the importance of strategies to defend against stressful situations and teaches specific coping strategies. Assisting individuals to consider the stressors in their lives and strategies to reduce them is an important aspect of pain management.

Cognitive errors

A number of cognitive errors in thinking have been associated with chronic pain (Melzack and Wall, 1982, 1996). These include dichotomous black-and-white reasoning, catastrophization, selective abstraction, personalization, overgeneralization and arbitrary reference (see Beck, 1976, for descriptions). Cognitive errors are thought to represent a maladaptive cognitive interpretation of pain (Turk and Rudy, 1988). This exacerbates, attenuates, maintains and distorts the experience of pain and suffering (Turk, 1994). These errors are linked to depression (Jensen et al., 1987; Philips, 1989; Smith, Peck and Ward, 1990; Sullivan and D'Eton, 1990;

Slater et al., 1991), severity (Flor and Turk, 1988) and disability (Flor and Turk, 1988; Smith et al., 1988). The cognitive errors that people make are explored in PMPs as part of an understanding of the role of unhelpful thinking. Individuals are encouraged to identify and challenge them.

Strategies to improve coping

Current PMPs emphasize coping rather than cure. Coping is regarded as the effort the individual makes to manage and minimize negative experiences. PMPs help this process of managing and minimizing negative experience by teaching strategies.

Strategies typically included in cognitive–behavioural PMPs are divided into those that modify pain-related cognitions and those aimed at modifying cognitive responses to stress (Meichenbaum, 1977; Turk and Genest, 1979). Strategies taught might include a number of the following (Tan, 1982):

- *Imaginative inattention.* Individuals are taught how to relax and imagine themselves in an environment that is safe, pleasant and incompatible with the pain – such as lying on a beach.
- *Imaginative transformation of pain.* Sensations associated with the pain are given different labels such as tingling, tightness, numbness and cold.
- *Imaginative transformation of context.* Pain is acknowledged but the context in which it occurs is changed. An example might be carrying a heavy child out of danger. Bravery rather than fear becomes an associated emotion.
- *Attention diversion.* Attention is directed to other things such as counting backwards, or using environmental cues such as counting ceiling tiles.
- *Somatization.* Attention is turned onto the pain but in a detached manner, focusing on bodily changes and sensations.

Tan (1982) analysed 27 studies that had taught a variety of cognitive strategies. Fifteen indicated that these strategies were superior to those generated by the individual themselves. The other 12 studies failed to demonstrate significant differences, suggesting that they may not all be helpful to all individuals. Chaves and Barber (1974) identified a number of individuals in their study who would have preferred to use their own strategies. This may reflect individuals' different beliefs and attributional style (Buchanan and Seligman, 1995) and, accordingly, require different strategies (Williams and Keefe, 1991) and imaginative flexibility when helping people to consider alternatives.

Control

Coping strategies are regarded as playing a significant role in changing beliefs that individuals hold about the degree of control they have and as a consequence help to improve their self-efficacy. Both control and self-efficacy have been found to be important aspects in pain perception.

The concept of locus of control (Rotter, 1966) refers to the beliefs that individuals have about whether outcomes are under their control (internal locus of control) or controlled by things other than themselves (external locus of control). Beliefs about control have been found to exert significant influence on behaviours, thoughts and feelings. Harakapaa et al. (1991) found that, of 476 individuals with chronic lower back pain, those who had an internal locus of control and used exercise regimens were less disabled on the completion of either inpatient or outpatient PMPs. Skevington (1983) identified that people with chronic back pain were more likely to be depressed and distressed by their pain if they believed events happened because of chance. A study by Turk, Rudy and Kerns (1988) investigated the relationship between perceived locus of control and perceived interference of pain and depression. Both external locus of control and high perceived interference increased the likelihood of depression and influenced the relationship between pain severity and depression. Sullivan and D'Eton (1990) found that the more individuals believed in personal control the less likely they were to regard the pain as interfering with their lives.

However, it is not clear whether PMPs increase a measure of internal control and hence change pain or whether a reduction in pain enables internal control to be regained.

Self-efficacy

Self-efficacy theory (Bandura, 1977) maintains that change, whether behavioural or cognitive, relates to people's beliefs about their ability to gain mastery. This concept is important for PMPs, as a degree of mastery over the pain is a primary objective. An increase in self-efficacy is considered to occur through the processes of improving coping strategies, understanding and implementing changes in the interactions of thoughts, feelings, behaviour, physical reactions and environment.

A study by Bandura et al. (1987) assessed perceived self-efficacy and pain control in a laboratory experiment. It demonstrated that cognitive strategy training increased perceived self-efficacy and the ability of the individual to endure and alleviate pain.

Increasing self-efficacy in PMPs has not been satisfactorily demonstrated, although Schiaffino, Revenson and Gibofsky (1991) showed that strong self-efficacy beliefs were associated with greater problem solving, coping and less disability a year later.

Family dynamics

Increasingly PMPs involve family members at some stage. The foundations of this are partly related to the influence of behavioural therapy and partly due to the increasing understanding of the function of family dynamics on the pain experience. Roy (1986: 113) states that even a 'well-functioning family, can, in a very short space of time, become almost totally dysfunctional when one of its members assumes the role of a chronic pain patient'. Research evidence indicates the significant role that families can have on perpetuating and prolonging the pain experience (Block, Kremer and Gaylor, 1980; Roy 1982). Changes in roles, interpersonal relationships, financial burdens, emotional support, sexual gratification, and disability and family activities are also identified as reasons to involve family members.

Summary

The above highlights the variety of different elements that contribute to a PMP. The elements range from increasing physical activity to evaluating and considering the interaction of thoughts, feelings, behaviour, physical responses and the environment. Each element has found its place in the PMP process through, paradoxically, both poor and improved understanding.

Relationships

A failure to provide and understand why a pain-free existence for all individuals is not currently possible has challenged both conceptualization and treatment of pain. While cure remains elusive a difference can be made in the lives of chronic pain sufferers by taking a holistic and respectful view of them and their situation.

Through working with individuals in chronic pain the author's experience is that PMPs can be in danger of becoming the ubiquitous 'pill' for those individuals who cannot be managed by medication and have become challenging to the medical profession. They appear to be used as the last staging post rather than a crucial early holistic response. Most significantly, the biopsychosocial approach is rarely adopted and used outside of these programmes, even within pain clinics, which often makes it extremely difficult to break cycles of dysfunction even when someone has attended a PMP.

The doctor and 'patient' have a relationship that is a social process large-ly defined by the role expectations each occupies. At a simplistic level this is to cure (the doctor) and be cured (the patient). However, there are only a certain number of available options with which to attempt this expected cure (think elephant and specialist). During acute stages of pain the expectation on both sides is likely to be relatively realistic and in most cases pain is permanently and effectively alleviated. However, as pain becomes chronic, the doctor's and the patient's expectations are challenged increasingly.

Eventually chronic pain sufferers begin to realize that the doctor is not tak-ing their pain away. As a consequence they appear either to become disillusioned with the medical profession or to continue to 'collect' both doc-tors and medication. In both cases it is probable that the role expectations held about doctors are challenged and the limitations of their profession dis-covered. Taylor (1979) describes two different behavioural/emotional repertoires of the patient who has had many hospital admissions and proce-dures. There is the angry, demanding, critical and suspicious individual who becomes known as the 'bad patient'. In comparison there is the passive, inan-imate and highly compliant individual who is regarded as a 'good patient'. It is possible that, as patients' role expectations change regarding the doctor's ability to cure their pain, they also begin to adopt one of these two positions with all the associated unhelpful and helpful consequences.

Equally, in this social process the doctor is likely to be confronted by his or her own fallibility and limitations as patients appear time and time again with little change in their presentation. It is the experience of the author that both the 'good' and the 'bad' patients present a challenge for the doc-tor. Part of this challenge is managing the internal dissonance that is generated by not being able to fulfil a fundamental role expectation, which is to be able to cure and 'make better'. As a consequence doctors appear to use every available intervention, both pharmaceutical and surgical, at their disposal in order to:

- 'dispose' of the patient who inadvertently creates the emotional dis-comfort;
- maintain the expectation that they can cure.

The reality, however, is that there are only so many options available to doc-tors if they retain a medical model as the single point of reference with respect to pain. The typical chronic pain sufferer eventually exhausts these. The development of PMPs has increased the options available and has pro-vided an opportunity to break the cycle for both the doctor and the patient by acknowledging that to cure and to be cured is not possible. However, the lead up to attending a PMP is often a long and drawn-out process where neither side appears able to accept and acknowledge that a 'cure' is not the solution.

The view of the PMP as the ubiquitous pill and last resort is in some ways unfortunate, destroying many things such as trust and belief in healthcare. However, it is the author's opinion that, unless things change dramatically in the social process between doctor and 'patient' and a biopsychosocial approach is adopted from the outset, it is unlikely that 'patients' would be able to let go of a belief that they can be pain free sooner.

The search for a pain-free existence and a label that makes sense of the pain are important to people. Uncertainty is an uncomfortable position to occupy – especially when people have no idea how long something is going to last and the outcome is ambiguous. This is likely to be an experience shared by both the clinician and the sufferer. Viney (1983) identified six significant emotions associated with severe illness where anxiety, anger and denial were common themes. Also noted was that uncertainty and not knowing increased people's general levels of vulnerability and helplessness. Skevington (1995) suggests that the ambiguous meaning of a person's illness is constantly being negotiated in a dynamic process where meaning is constructed even in the absence of not knowing.

In many respects the social process between the doctor and patient role expectations becomes a grieving process in which individuals begin to acknowledge and accept their losses so that they can move forward from the position of 'a person in *chronic pain*' to being a '*person* with chronic pain'. This is a necessary and emotionally painful journey (nearly always, in the author's view, reflected in the person's physical pain experience) towards an acceptance that they may always be in chronic pain and that they need to find alternative ways of coping and opening new avenues in their lives.

Summary

The consequences of chronic pain are far reaching and affect all relationships that chronic pain sufferers have and the relationship that others have with them. The impact of meeting someone who is in excruciating, unrelenting pain and whose suffering is so apparent can leave everyone feeling helpless and stuck.

Individual stories

AD

AD's experience during the PMP was certainly very challenging. Following the assessment it was left to him to consider whether to join the group and it took a number of weeks for him to reach the decision to do so. As he turned the corner he established some good life-changing goals, paced himself, and considered his thinking patterns. He also shifted from being in a constant rage with the world to a more relaxed and comfortable position where he could take his time and let go of some of his need to always be in control. He is still in pain, he takes no medication and is doing more now than he has done in 7 years.

JS

JS is a 50-year-old woman who, in 1987, was involved in a road traffic accident. A year and a day later she was operated on following a radiculogram (also known as a myelogram), which showed she had two herniated discs. The year between the accident and surgery had been torturous, not only due to the severity of her pain but also because of her experience that no one was listening to her. For approximately 3 years she was relatively pain free but gradually the pain 'sneaked back'. It was considered to be caused by scar tissue near the sciatic nerve.

Prior to the accident, JS worked and trained racehorses. The pain prevented her from continuing with this and she had not ridden a horse since because she did not think she could or should. She was working long hours as a cleaner and had identified that the days she did not work the pain was less bearable. She had adapted to her pain by not letting anyone know and made jokes constantly about herself in order to cover up her vulnerability. JS was determined not to let the pain impact too greatly on her life even before coming on the course and in many respects she had found her own strategies of how to manage the pain. However, the strategies generally involved 'being stoical' and just getting on with it. She did not believe she had the right to identify and consider her own needs; she felt unable to say 'no' and regarded herself as useless if she stopped even for a rest. She was taking a cocktail of medication including co-proxamol, amitriptyline and caffeine.

During the PMP she was an important member providing light relief and compassion for others. She is a carer and often deflected others' care for her away with a joke or by dismissing their observations, particularly those that were complimentary. During the course she learned how to take care of herself more and how her joking acted as a deflection and a defence. She recognized that sometimes it was necessary for her to joke things away but other times this prevented people from taking care of her. She learned that saying 'no' was all right and that nothing major would happen as a consequence. She slowed down to a degree but was never able to stop taking the medication, partly, I think, because she continued to work at an extremely hard rate.

Although she still works at a high rate she now changes what she is doing so she is not in one position for hours on end (she used to iron for at least 3 hours without a break). She also recognizes her limitations and does not try to move wardrobes on her own any longer! She discovered that she can ask for help and that this does not mean she is a lesser person.

JS very quickly took to relaxation and she continues, 3 years after the course, to listen to her relaxation tape every night. Her greatest discovery was how she had let her pain defeat her, making her believe she could not do the things she enjoyed. She has recently ridden a horse again.

She says that meeting other people was the most important aspect of the PMP. In the PMP setting she did not feel she had to prove herself to anyone. She had always felt that she needed to prove she could still do things even though, paradoxically, she had given so much up. The degree of control she gave to others was actually quite high. This was reflected in her thinking not only about what she should or should not do but also in the levels of expectation she held. She had to be 'good' rather than 'good enough'.

JS remains in pain and what the PMP offered her regarding her pain managing strategies was limited. However she took an enormous amount away, which improved her self-respect, and her ability to relax and define her own parameters. She was able to use the assertiveness and communication elements of the PMP to good effect. Her activity levels outside work increased and she no longer bars herself from doing things that she thinks she would enjoy.

JAS

JAS is a 30-year-old mother of two. Two years after the birth of her second child she bent over and pulled out a bed, hurting her lower back. This initial pain eased over time but returned 6 months later. A cyclical pattern developed where JAS was in some pain, although not excruciating pain, but was then in severe pain for a period of time. The medications she took included co-proxamol, co-dydramol and diazepam and, at the time we met, she had also been on antidepressants for a number of months.

The time between the pain developing and our meeting was approximately 3 years. In this time she describes herself as having become more and more isolated and doing less and less. The depression she was feeling had increased to the degree that she felt that life was not worth living. Her pain had escalated beyond a cyclical pattern so that she was now experiencing constant and disabling pain. JAS's husband was largely responsible for doing the household chores, which served to increase her sense of worthlessness.

She had met with the pain anaesthetist a number of times prior to her referral to a PMP. However, she felt increasingly that the painkillers were not helping and that no one knew what was causing the pain. This intensified a feeling of despondency and hopelessness as she struggled with an increasing sense that her life was going to consist of her being constantly in pain and dependent upon other people. At the time the PMP came up she felt at her most desperate and she was willing to try anything. As a consequence of this desperation she did not experience any difficulty with the thought that she was being sent to meet with a clinical psychologist. During the course of the assessment she began to recognize the possibility that her pain experience could relate to her mood, her view of herself and her life at that time. JAS was open and receptive to the biopsychosocial model.

At the outset of the course JAS felt like a fraud because she perceived the other participants as more extreme in their disability. However, she rapidly recognized the similarities and that they understood how she was feeling. The sense of shared experience and understanding was an important factor for JAS.

She was a valuable member of the group because she was able to consider and work with the models being presented. She was able to recognize the interrelationship of her thoughts, feelings and behaviour and the impact on her pain experience. For a time she struggled with the thinking element but patiently worked with it and diligently recorded her experiences in order to bring them back to the group and consider the relationships. Both her mood and pain improved during the course. Eventually she felt able to apply for a job. With the encouragement of the group she applied, was interviewed and has been working for several years.

As JAS says, setbacks happened and they were extremely hard to cope with after the course had finished as she felt back on her own again. However, she has continued to refer back to the manual that charted the PMP elements. She has continued with her relaxation and exercises and is acutely aware that her pain links intimately with the emotional stress she is experiencing in her life.

She regards the reappearance of her pain as a form of communication and feels that she needs to listen to it by considering what in her life is problematic and disturbing her. By doing this she has found herself able to address the 'real' cause of the pain with the result that the pain rapidly dissipates and she can move on again.

JAS's case illustrates that, on the surface, some people's experience of chronic pain can appear to be physiological. While it is highly probable that physical injury occurred initially, it has long since resolved and the pain has taken on a meaning and function in the individual's life. She has learned to recognize the meaning of her pain and that it relates more to how she is feeling psychologically than physically. She also now knows that if she does not address the psychological issues the pain increases and she begins to feel low. The vicious cycle is then more in danger of becoming entrenched and the control slips away from her and towards the pain.

Conclusion

Turk (1994: 45) states that pain 'involves conscious awareness, selective abstraction, appraisal, ascribed meaning, and learning'. It 'is best viewed as a perceptual and not purely sensory process'. This view is a significant departure from a purely sensory understanding of pain and has emerged from attempts to understand the factors that contribute to the complex ways that pain and chronic pain present.

Different conceptual models have been found to be useful in helping both theoretical understanding of the development of pain into a chronic condition and clinical treatment. It is necessary to identify scientifically driven conceptual theories and models not only to symbolically represent what is known but also to improve understanding by testing the predictions made by the models.

Theories and models that regard pain as more than a purely sensory experience include the biopsychosocial model, gate-control theory and cognitive–behavioural theory. The generic biopsychosocial model has been highlighted as a powerful and necessary approach in understanding, assessing and treating chronic pain. This model has been found to be extremely useful and appropriate as it supports the evidence suggesting that chronic pain is not a linear bottom-up sensory dysfunction. Using the model as a holistic approach ensures consideration of chronic pain as something that is derived from and maintained by a range of potentially contributing factors that interrelate in a complex manner. This can then incorporate understanding offered by theories and models from other disciplines.

Multidisciplinary PMPs are continuing to develop and inform understanding. They are highly structured and complex. They begin a process of reconceptualizing the problems that people are experiencing and offer alternatives to an expectation of a pain-free existence. This process should occur at an earlier stage than it often does and clinicians from all disciplines should be more familiar with current understanding about pain and the factors that contribute to its development into a chronic state with all the consequent suffering.

References

Bandura A (1977) Self-efficacy: toward a unifying theory of behavioural change. Psychological Review 84: 191–215.

Bandura A, O'Leary A, Taylor C et al. (1987) Perceived self-efficacy and pain control: opioid and nonopioid mechanisms. Journal of Personality and Social Psychology 3: 563–71.

Banks S, Kerns R (1996) Explaining high rates of depression in chronic pain: a diathesis-stress framework. Psychological Bulletin 119: 95–110.

Beck A (1976) Cognitive Therapy and Emotional Disorders. London: Penguin.

Beecher H (1956) Relationship of significance of wound to pain experienced. Journal of the American Medical Association 161: 1609–13.

Beecher H (1960) Increased stress and effectiveness of placebos and activity drugs. Science 132: 91–2.

Blanchard E, Theobold D, Williamson D et al. (1978) Temperature biofeedback in the treatment of migraine headaches. Archives of General Psychiatry 35: 581–8.

Block A, Kremer E, Gaylor M (1980) Behavioural treatment of chronic pain: the spouse as a discriminative cue for pain behaviour. Pain 9: 243–52.

Bonica JJ (ed.) (1990) History of pain concepts and therapies. In The Management of Pain. Philadelphia PA: Lee & Febiger.

Buchanan G, Seligman M (1995) Explanatory Style. Hillside, NY: Erlbaum.

Cairns D, Thomas L, Mooney V et al. (1976) A comprehensive treatment approach to chronic low back pain. Pain 2: 301–8.

Chaves J, Barber T (1974) Cognitive strategies, experimenter modelling and expectation in the attention of pain. Journal of Abnormal Psychology 83: 356–63.

Cox D, Freundlich A, Meyer R (1975) Differential effectiveness of electromyograph feedback, verbal relaxation instructions and medication placebo with tension headaches. Pain 43: 892–8.

Eccleston C, Williams AC, Rogers WS (1997) Patients 'and professionals' understanding of the causes of chronic pain: blame, responsibility and identity protection. Social Science and Medicine 45: 699–709.

Edwards L, Pearce S, Turner-Stokes L, Jones A (1992) The pain beliefs questionnaire: an investigation of beliefs in the causes and consequences of pain patients. Pain 51: 267–72.

Elliott AM, Smith BH, Hannaford PC, Smith WC, Chambers WA (2002) The course of chronic pain in the community: results of a 4-year follow-up study. Pain 99(1–2): 299–307.

Fernadez E, Turk D (1992) Sensory and affective components of pain: separation and synthesis. Psychological Bulletin 112: 205–17.

Flor H, Turk D (1988) Chronic back pain and rheumatoid arthritis: predicting pain and disability from cognitive variables. Journal of Behavioural Medicine 11(3): 251–65.

Flor H, Turk D (1989) Psychophysiology of chronic pain: do chronic pain patients exhibit symptom-specific psychophysiological responses? Psychological Bulletin 105: 215–59.

Fordyce W (1976) Behavioural Methods in Chronic Pain and Illness. St Louis, MO: Mosby.

Fordyce W, Fowler R, Lehmann J et al. (1968) Some implications of learning in problems of chronic pain. Journal of Chronic Diseases 21: 179–90.

Fordyce W, Fowler R, Lehmann J et al. (1973) Operant conditioning in the treatment of chronic pain. Archives of Physical and Medical Rehabilitation 54: 399–408.

Fordyce W, Roberts A, Sternbach R (1985) The behavioural management of chronic pain: a response to the critics. Pain 22: 113–25.

Gallagher R (1999) Treatment planning in pain medicine. Intergrating medical, physical and behavioural therapies. Medical Clinics of North America 83: 823–49.

Gallagher R, McCann WJ, Jerman A et al (1990) The behavioural medicine service – an administrative model for biopsychosocial medical care, teaching and research. General Hospital Psychiatry 12: 283–95.

Gamsa A (1990) Is emotional disturbance a precipitator or a consequence of chronic pain? Pain 42: 183–95.

Gamsa A (1994) The role of psychological factors in chronic pain. I. A half century of study. Pain 57: 5–15.

Gentry W, Owen D (1986) Pain groups. In Holzman A, Turk D (eds) Pain Management. A Handbook of Psychological Treatment Approaches. New York: Pergamon.

Greenberger D, Padesky C (1995) Mind Over Mood. Change How You Feel by Changing the Way You Think. New York: Guilford Press.

Harakapaa K, Jarvikoski A, Mellin G et al. (1991) Health locus of control beliefs and psychological distress as predictors for treatment outcomes in low back pain: patients' results of a three-month follow up of a controlled intervention study. Pain 46: 35–41.

Haynes S, Griffin P, Mooney D, Parise M (1975) Electromyographic biofeedback and relaxation instructions in the treatment of muscle contraction headaches. Behaviour Therapy 6: 672–8.

Hendler N (1981) Diagnostic and Nonsurgical Management of Chronic Pain. New York: Raven Press.

Herman E, Baptiste S (1981) Pain control: mastery through group experience. Pain 10: 79–86.

Jensen MP, Karoly P, Huger R (1987) The development and preliminary validation of an instrument to assess patients' attitudes towards pain. Journal of Psychosomatic Research 31(3): 393–400.

Karoly P (1985) Measurement Strategies in Health Psychology. New York: John Wiley & Sons.

Keefe F, Block A, Williams R et al. (1981) Behavioural treatment of chronic low back pain: clinical outcome and individual differences in pain relief. Pain 11(2): 221–31.

LaRocca H (1992) A taxonomy of chronic pain syndromes: 1991 presidential address, cervical spine research society annual meeting, December 5, 1991. Spine 17(10Supp): S344– 55.

Lethern J, Slade P, Troup J et al. (1983) Outline of a fear-avoidance model of exaggerated pain perception. Behaviour Research and Therapy 21(4): 401–8.

Linton SJ, Gotestarn KG (1984) A controlled study of the effects of applied relaxation and applied relaxation plus operant procedures in the regulation of chronic pain. The British Journal of Clinical Psychology 23(4): 291–9.

McCracken L, Zayfert C, Gross R (1992) The pain anxiety symptoms scale: development and validation of a scale to measure fear of pain. Pain 50: 67–73.

Meichenbaum D (1977) Cognitive Behaviour Modification. An Integrative Approach. New York: Plenum Publishing Corp.

Melzack R (1973) The Puzzle of Pain. New York: Basic Books.

Melzack R, Wall P (1965) Pain mechanisms: a new theory. Science 150: 971–9.

Melzack R, Wall P (1982, 1988, 1996) The Challenge of Pain. Harmondsworth: Penguin.

Merskey H (1985) A mentalistic view of pain and behaviour. Behaviour, Brain and Science 8: 65.

Nicholas MK, Wilson P, Goyen J (1992) Comparison of cognitive behavioural group treatment and an alternative non-psychological treatment for chronic low back pain. Pain 48(3): 339–47.

Pain Society (1997) Report of a Working Party of The Pain Society of Great Britain and Northern Ireland. The British, Irish Chapter of the International Association for the Study of Pain. London: The Pain Society.

Philips HC (1989) Thoughts provoked by pain. Behaviour Research Therapy 27(4): 469–73.

Roberts A, Reinhardt L (1980) The behavioural management of chronic pain: Long term follow up with comparison groups. Pain 8(2): 151–62.

Rotter JB (1966) Generalized expectancies for internal versus external reinforcement of control. Psychological Monographs 80(1): 1–28.

Roy R (1982) Marital and family issues in chronic pain. Psychotherapy and Psychosomatics 37(1): 1–12.

Roy R (1985) The interactional perspective of pain behaviour in marriage. International Journal of Family Therapy 7: 271–82.

Roy R (1986) A family systems approach. In Holzam A, Turk D (eds) Pain Management. A Handbook of Psychological Treatment Approaches. New York: Pergamon

Schiaffino KM, Revenson T, Gibofsky A (1991) Assessing the impact of self efficacy beliefs on adaptation to rheumatoid arthritis. Arthritis Care and Research 4(4): 150–7.

Schmidt A (1987) The behavioural management of pain: a criticism of a response. Pain 30(3): 285–91.

Sheehan G (1994) Thoughts about exercise. Baillière's Clinical Rheumatology 8(1): 1–5.

Skevington SM (1983) Chronic pain and depression: universal or personal helplessness. Pain 15(3): 309–17.

Skevington S (1995) Psychology of Pain. New York: Wiley.

Skinner BJ, Erskine A, Pearce S et al. (1990) The evaluation of a cognitive behavioural treatment programme in outpatients with chronic pain. Journal of Psychosomatic Research 34(1): 13–19.

Slater M, Hall H, Atkinson J et al. (1991) Pain and impairment beliefs in chronic low back pain: Validation of the pain and impairment relationship scale (PAIRS). Pain 44: 51–6.

Smith T, Peck J, Miliano R, Ward J (1988) Cognitive distortion in rheumatoid arthritis: relation to depression and disability. Journal of Consulting and Clinical Psychology 56: 412–16.

Smith T, Peck J, Ward J (1990) Helplessness and depression in rheumatoid arthritis. Health Psychology 9: 377–89.

Sullivan M, D'Eton J (1990) Relation between catastrophizing and depression in chronic pain patients. Journal of Abnormal Psychology 99: 260–3.

Tan S (1982) Cognitive and cognitive behavioural methods for pain control: a selective review. Pain 12: 201–28.

Taylor S (1979) Hospital patient behaviour: reactance, helplessness or control? Journal of Social Issues 35: 156–84.

Tuke D (1884) Illustrations of the Influence of the Mind Upon the Body in Health and Disease Designed to Elucidate the Imagination, 2nd edn. Philadelphia, PA: Henry Lea's.

Turk D (1994) Perspectives on chronic pain: the role of psychological factors. Current Directions in Psychological Science 3: 45–8.

Turk D, Flor H (1984) Etiological theories and treatments for chronic back pain. II. Psychological models–interventions. Pain 19: 209–33.

Turk D, Genest M (1979) Regulation of pain. The application of cognitive and behavioural techniques for prevention and remediation. In Kendall P, Hollon S (eds) Cognitive Behavioural Interventions: Theory, Research and Procedures. New York: Academic Press.

Turk D, Rudy T (1983) Cognitive factors and persistent pain. A glimpse in Pandora's box. Cognitive Therapy and Research 16: 99–122.

Turk D, Rudy T, Kerns R (1988) Chronic pain and depression: towards a cognitive behavioural mediation model. Pain 35: 129–40.

Turner J (1991) Coping and chronic pain. In Bond M, Charlton J, Woolf C (eds) Proceedings of the VIth World Congress on Pain. Amsterdam: Elsevier.

Turner J, Chapman C (1982) Psychological interventions for chronic pain: a critical review 1. Relaxation training and biofeedback. Pain 12: 1–21.

Viney LL (1983) Images of Illness. Malabar, FL: Kreiger.

Wall P, Melzack R (1983) Textbook of Pain. Edinburgh: Churchill Livingstone.

Weiner B (1985) An attributional theory of achievement, motivation and emotion. Psychological Review 92: 548–75.

Weir R, Woodside D, Crook J (1988) Group therapy for chronic pain patients: a view of the complexity. Pain Clinic 2: 109–20.

Williams D, Keefe F (1991) Pain beliefs and the use of cognitive behavioural coping strategies. Pain 46: 185–219.

CHAPTER TWO

Physiology of chronic pain

MARK JOHNSON

Aim

To introduce the concepts that underpin the physiological mechanisms contributing to clinical pain. In order to ascribe physiological mechanisms to pain it is important to analyse the nature of pain itself.

Objectives

At the end of this chapter the reader will:

- have an understanding of the processes involved in pain transmission;
- be aware of different types of pain.

Introduction

In 1992, the International Association for the Study of Pain (IASP) Task Force for Acute Pain concluded that healthcare professionals without sufficient knowledge on the physiology of pain were more likely to give a low priority to pain treatment because of the misguided belief that hurting is normal and harmless (Ready and Edwards, 1992). If healthcare professionals are also overfearful of addiction or respiratory depression associated with giving opioid analgesics like morphine, patients are likely to receive insufficient analgesia (Cousins and Power, 1999). Patients in pain experience a variety of physiological changes that can be detrimental to their health such as increased blood pressure, altered blood gases, delayed gastric emptying, urinary retention and the production of 'stress hormones' (Figure 2.1). It is important to manage the patient's pain appropriately to reduce the incidence and severity of these adverse physiological effects.

Interestingly, healthcare professionals often find the experience of learning about pain physiology painful! One reason for this could be the level of attention given to physiological and pharmacological minutiae in the literature, leaving readers with an overwhelming sense of incomprehensible complexity. Healthcare professionals need to know the basic physiological concepts that underpin symptoms and response to treatment, rather than physiological minutiae, so that they can make informed clinical decisions and actions.

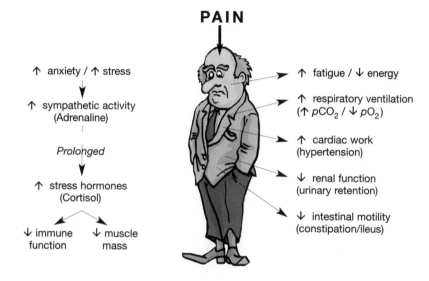

PAIN

↑ anxiety / ↑ stress

↓

↑ sympathetic activity
(Adrenaline)

Prolonged

↓

↑ stress hormones
(Cortisol)

↓ immune   ↓ muscle
function   mass

↑ fatigue / ↓ energy

↑ respiratory ventilation
($\uparrow pCO_2$ / $\downarrow pO_2$)

↑ cardiac work
(hypertension)

↓ renal function
(urinary retention)

↓ intestinal motility
(constipation/ileus)

Figure 2.1 Physiological response to pain.

The nature of pain

Defining pain

The word 'pain' is used to describe unpleasant sensations that are often associated with injury to the body. However, most sensory experiences are difficult to describe; try to explain the difference between the colour blue and red to a person who has never been able to see. Sensations are personal experiences and we learn to use certain words to try to convey these experiences to others so that a shared understanding of the meaning of these words develops in society. An accurate definition is 'pain is what the patient says it is' because we can only be confident that a sensory experience is painful when a person uses the word 'pain' to describe it. Consequently, the assessment of a patient's pain is related to patients' ability to articulate exactly what it is they are experiencing. Words like 'shooting', 'stabbing', 'aching', 'lanciating' are often used to describe the characteristics and nature of pain. They are often accompanied by words that convey our feelings about pain like 'distressing', 'uncomfortable' and 'annoying'. Our ability to select and use such words depends on our previous experience of pain and on the use of the words by others around us. A wide variety of factors may influence the words used by patients to describe pain experience such as gender, culture and environmental setting (Melzack, 1975; Melzack and Katz, 1999).

The IASP defines pain as: 'an unpleasant sensory and emotional experience associated with actual or potential tissue damage, or described in terms of such damage' (Merskey, 1986, 1991). This definition highlights that pain can be produced without actual tissue damage (by potential tissue damage) and that pain has sensory and emotional dimensions to it.

Dimensions of pain

Pain is often described in terms of sensory, affective (emotional) and cognitive (thinking) dimensions (Figure 2.2) (Melzack and Katz, 1999). The sensory dimensions of pain relate to the intensity, location and quality of the pain, and are sub-served by neural circuitry that is called the nociceptive system. The nociceptive system has evolved to detect events (i.e. stimuli) in our internal and external environment that are noxious (noci) and have the potential to produce tissue damage. When noxious stimuli are detected the nociceptive system elicits behaviours that attempt to reduce the impact of tissue damage on the body, such as withdrawal reflexes and escape responses (Figure 2.3).

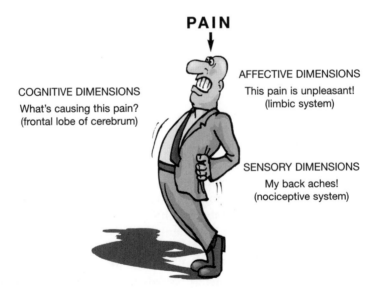

Figure 2.2 The dimensions of pain.

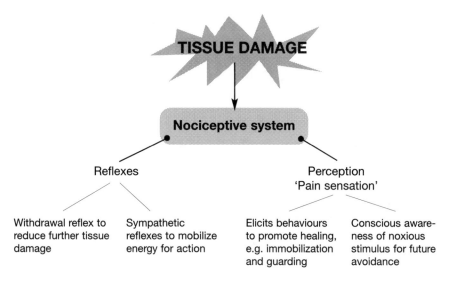

Figure 2.3 Responses elicited by the nociceptive system.

The nociceptive system can generate a sensory experience that we learn to recognize as pain so that we become consciously aware of the noxious stimuli.

All sensations (for example, touch, vision, hearing, taste and smell) are generated by neural activity in the higher centres of the brain and not by the body parts that detect the stimulus. This is clearly observed when a limb is severed from a person's body and that person can no longer feel someone else touching the severed limb because the neural connections between the limb and brain have been broken. It was thought that the somatosensory cortex of the cerebrum of the brain would generate the intensity, location and quality of pain because it receives neural input from the surface of the body (for example, the skin). This somatic ('body parts') input arrives from the opposite side of the body (contralateral) and in an ordered fashion (Figure 2.4). Each somatic structure can be mapped across the surface of the somatosensory cortex to form a homunculus ('little man') (Penfield, 1968). Sensitive parts of the body such as the hands and face have proportionately larger areas of the cortex devoted to processing incoming information compared with less sensitive areas such as the trunk. The area of the somatosensory cortex devoted to processing incoming information is related to the density of sensory receptor cells in the body part. However, it has been found that the removal of inputs to the somatosensory cortex, or removal of the somatosensory cortex itself, does not appear to alter pain in the long term in humans (Tasker, 1994; Gybels and Tasker, 1999; Ingvar and Hsieh, 1999; Treede et al., 2000). This suggests that the somatosensory cortex does not generate the sensory dimensions of pain as such and that the physiological mechanisms involved are more complex than first thought.

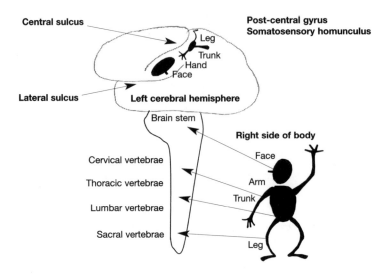

Figure 2.4 Somatotopic ('body map') representation in the central nervous system. Somatosensory receptors send information into the central nervous system at given segments of the spinal cord, forming a dermatomal map. Somatosensory pathways in the central nervous system project in an ordered fashion to given areas of the contralateral somatosensory cortex. Large areas of the somatosensory cortex are given over to processing input from body parts that have fine discrimination creating a distorted body map termed a 'homunculus'.

The affective dimensions of pain relate to emotions and feelings associated with pain and are described using words like distress, unpleasant, discomfort, annoying and terrifying. The limbic system, which is often considered to be the 'emotional centre' of the brain, contains structures such as the amygdala, hippocampus and cingulate gyrus (Figure 2.5). The cingulate gyrus plays a crucial role in the affective dimensions of pain as demonstrated in brain imaging studies and in surgical techniques such as cingulotomy which reduce the emotional aspects of patients' pain (Gybels and Tasker, 1999; Ingvar and Hsieh, 1999). The cognitive dimensions of pain relate to thoughts associated with pain and involve analysing the cause of the pain and determining the most appropriate behaviour to remove the pain. The frontal lobe of the cerebral cortex is likely to be involved in generating cognitive dimensions of pain.

The relative contribution of sensory, affective and cognitive dimensions to pain varies according to an individual's situation. Patients with pain of known cause and short duration, such as post-surgical pain, are likely to have fewer affective and cognitive contributions to their pain when compared with patients with long-standing pain of unknown cause. Thus, approaches to pain management must be flexible and multidisciplinary.

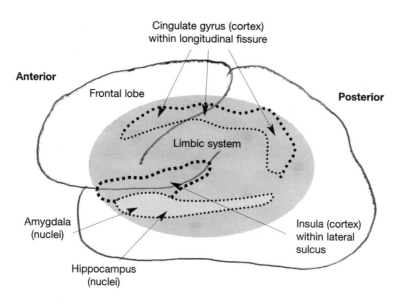

Figure 2.5 Areas of the cerebrum involved in affective and cognitive dimensions of pain. The limbic system comprises many regions of cerebral cortex and subcortical nuclei that are implicated in the affective dimensions of pain. The frontal lobe plays a crucial role in thought processing and is likely to contribute to the cognitive dimensions of pain.

Pain and injury

The IASP definition states that pain may arise from actual or potential tissue damage and this suggests that the link between pain and injury may be variable. Observations support this premise (Figure 2.6):

- Pain despite considerable tissue damage, as seen when military personnel request no analgesic medication following traumatic battlefield injury. In this situation pain seems to have been suppressed.
- Pain when movements are made that normally do not produce pain, as seen when walking on a twisted ankle. In this situation, pain seems to have been exaggerated or amplified.
- Pain that persists beyond the normal time expected for the injury to heal, as seen in phantom limb pain, which persists despite the healing of the original damage in the stump of the amputated limb. In this situation pain seems to occur in the absence of ongoing tissue damage.
- Pain in body parts that differ from the site of injury, as seen in patients experiencing pain down the left arm during a myocardial infarction. In this situation pain seems to be referred to another part of the body.
- Pain that is out of proportion to the injury, as seen when a sliver of metal embeds itself under a fingernail to produce excruciating pain.

- In contrast, tissue damage that is life threatening, such as a large malignant tumour, may go unnoticed. In these situations pain appears to vary according to different body tissues and structures.

These examples demonstrate that the relationship between pain and injury is not always predictable and depends to some extent on circumstance.

The analysis of the nature of pain has shown that pain is not a unitary phenomenon. It is likely that a variety of physiological mechanisms will contribute to the different aspects of pain described in this section. In many respects, the notion of a 'pain system' that is both multidimensional and dynamic has only recently been accepted.

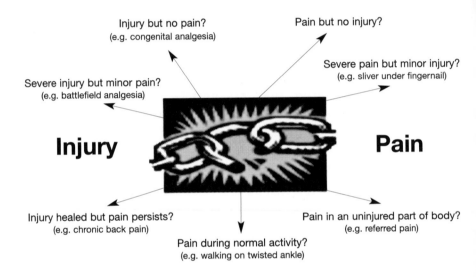

Figure 2.6 The variable link between pain and injury.

The physiology of pain: evolution of knowledge

Physiological knowledge can change with time so that what is believed to be a 'fact' today may well be dispelled as 'fiction' in the future. Once fiction is accepted as 'fact' it proves very difficult to reverse. In addition, physiological concepts have to be simplified for general consumption and this can lead to misrepresentation of information. Ultimately medical knowledge exists with a certain amount of instability.

Specificity theory

Over 300 years ago, Descartes suggested that there was a physiological system specifically dedicated to generating the sensation of pain. The theory implied that the pain system would faithfully reproduce pain whenever it was activated by an injury to the body. The specificity theory had an enormous impact in physiology, becoming the mainstay of many medical textbooks and having a marked effect on the approaches used to manage pain. Approaches like cutting 'pain pathways' using cordotomies, rhizotomies and cortical ablations became popular but were found to provide limited long-lasting pain relief. Clinical observations of patients in pain also suggested that the link between pain and injury was more variable than allowed for in the specificity theory.

The pattern theory of pain

This theory offered an alternative and for many years competed with the specificity theory for acceptance. The pattern theory suggested that sensations were coded in the frequency (rate) of nerve impulses travelling in 'non-specific nerve pathways'. As the intensity of a stimulus increased, more nerve impulses would be produced resulting in stronger and stronger sensations until pain was finally produced. Nowadays, a combination of specificity and pattern mechanisms is believed to contribute to pain sensation.

The central summation theory of pain

In the 1940s the central summation theory of pain suggested that the central nervous system (CNS) played a role in amplifying input from peripheral systems so that weak stimuli such as light touch could, under certain circumstances, produce pain (Livingston, 1943). This theory helped to shift focus away from peripheral mechanisms contributing to pain and towards the role of the CNS. The suggestion in the 1950s that the CNS could also suppress incoming noxious information and reduce pain sensation (Noordenbos, 1959) paved the way for a seminal paper by Melzack and Wall (1965) often referred to as the gate-control theory of pain.

The gate-control theory of pain

This theory suggested that a metaphorical gate in the spinal cord regulated the flow of noxious information en route to higher centres in the CNS. If the gate were open, noxious information could reach the brain to generate a sensation of pain (Figure 2.7). If the gate were closed, noxious information could not reach the brain and a sensation of pain would not result. In physiological terms the 'gate' is synaptic junctions between neurons. Impulses arriving at the spinal cord in afferent fibres transmitting noxious events would open the gate by releasing excitatory neurotransmitters whereas impulses arriving at the spinal cord in afferent fibres transmitting non-noxious events would close the gate by releasing inhibitory neuro-transmitters. Moreover, impulses arriving at the spinal cord in pathways descending from the brain (descending pain inhibitory pathways) could also close the gate by releasing inhibitory neurotransmitters.

The gate-control theory of pain inspired a period of intense research into various ways of closing the 'pain gate' with techniques like trans-cutaneous electrical nerve stimulation (TENS), spinal cord stimulation, acupuncture and centrally acting drugs like opioids.

In recent decades attention has focused on the physiology and pharma-cology of hyperalgesia ('above pain') that accompanies tissue damage (Woolf, 1994). During hyperalgesia the nociceptive system becomes 'sensitive' to stimuli at both peripheral and central sites (termed peripheral and central sensitization respectively). Under normal circumstances the nociceptive sys-tem returns to its 'normal' pre-sensitized state once the injury heals, although this is far less likely to occur if there has been nerve damage. Persistent sensitization is likely to be a critical factor in some chronic pain conditions observed in clinical practice (Woolf and Salter, 2000). Normal, short-term sensitized and persistent sensitized states of pain appear to be closely related to the physiological mechanisms that contribute to transient, acute and chronic pain respectively (Melzack and Wall, 1988) and to physio-logical, inflammatory and neuropathic pain respectively (Woolf, 1987).

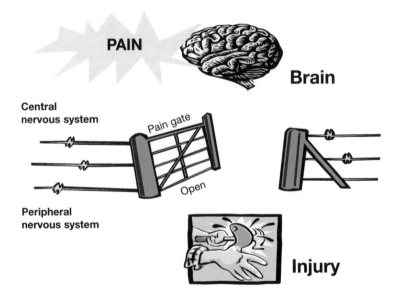

Figure 2.7 The 'pain gate'. Activity in nociceptive fibres, as generated by injury, opens the 'pain gate' so that it can access higher levels of the brain where it is processed to create a sensation of pain.

The neuromatrix theory of pain

This theory attempts to explain how pain sensations belong to the individual and has received much attention in the last decade (Melzack, 1990). It is claimed that the neuromatrix is a collection of neurons that are genetically predetermined to represent somatic structures and are modified throughout life according to the patterns of nerve activity elicited by everyday sensory stimuli. Nerve activity generated in the neuromatrix provides us with a flow of conscious awareness that we recognize as sensations that feel like they belong to ourselves. The neuromatrix theory of pain provides a plausible explanation for the symptoms of unusual conditions like phantom limb pain where pain occurs in limbs that no longer exist because of amputation. It is suggested that the neuromatrix tries to interpret the abnormal afferent input arising from nerves damaged by amputation and creates a phantom limb sensation.

At present, we know that pain is not a unitary phenomenon produced by a 'hard-wired' pain system but rather a dynamic sensation generated by a nociceptive system that can alter its sensitivity according to need and circumstance. Perhaps the easiest way to explore the physiological processes that produce pain is to consider brief transient pain, acute pain following tissue damage and persistent pain following the apparent healing of an injury. The mechanisms that produce these types of pain are sometimes called physiological pain, inflammatory (nociceptive) pain and neuropathic (pathophysiological) pain respectively (Woolf, 1987).

Types of pain

Transient, acute and chronic pain

Transient, acute and chronic pains are defined according to pain duration. Transient pain is defined as: 'Pain of brief duration and little consequence' (Melzack and Wall, 1988). It is the pain sensation that immediately follows a noxious event and usually consists of a sharp intense 'first' or 'fast' pain followed by a 'slow' or 'second' dull aching sensation (Table 2.1). If tissue damage is minimal (as when stubbing a toe, for example) the pain subsides quickly with no need for concern. Transient pain acts to prevent further injury by initiating escape and protective responses and by giving us an awareness of the type of stimuli that produce pain so that we can avoid them in the future. Humans rarely seek medical attention for transient pain resulting from minor accidents.

Acute pain is defined as: 'Pain of recent onset and probable limited duration. It usually has an identifiable temporal and causal relationship to injury and disease' (Ready and Edwards, 1992). Acute pain differs from transient pain because the stimulus generates appreciable tissue damage (Table 2.1). This results in physiological processes and behaviours that serve to promote healing, such as inflammation, tenderness and guarding behaviours to reduce additional damage to the injured body part. Often the injured area becomes sensitive to stimuli that hinder the repair of tissue, such as movement and touch. For example, when walking on a twisted ankle the pain sensation appears to be amplified so that walking produces pain and additional twisting of the ankle produces pain of much greater intensity than

Table 2.1 The characteristics of transient, acute and chronic pain

Characteristic	Transient	Acute	Chronic
Nature of primary 'pain' stimulus	Transitory noxious Potential tissue damage	Transitory noxious Actual tissue damage	Often unknown or persistent, ongoing tissue damage related to disease
Magnitude of initial pain sensation resulting from primary 'pain' stimulus	Often predictable Pain short-lived and of little consequence	Often predictable Pain related in magnitude and duration to the severity of the injury	Often no relationship May be predictable depending on disease
Sensations generated in response to subsequent stimuli	Normal Non-noxious stimuli produce non-noxious sensations (e.g. touch) Noxious stimuli produce pain	Amplified Non-noxious stimuli produce non-noxious sensations (e.g. touch) – allodynia Noxious stimuli produce exaggerated pain – hyperalgesia	Amplified Non-noxious stimuli produce non-noxious sensations (e.g. touch) – allodynia Noxious stimuli produce exaggerated pain – hyperalgesia
Physiological mechanisms	Nociceptive system activated	Nociceptive system activated with accompanying sensitization	Intractable sensitization due to pathophysiology in nociceptive system Nociceptive system continuously activated with accompanying sensitization
Function	Prevent tissue damage through escape responses Memory of noxious stimuli for future avoidance	Prevent further tissue damage through escape responses Promote healing through immobilization of injury	Maladaptive with no clear purpose Prevent further tissue damage to promote healing through immobilization of injury
Semantic correlates	Physiological pain Nociceptive pain	Nociceptive pain Inflammatory pain	Neuropathic pain Pathophysiological pain

normal. These symptoms of allodynia (tenderness) and hyperalgesia (exaggerated pain) are the result of the nociceptive system increasing its sensitivity to input from the periphery. Hyperalgesia is defined as: 'An increased response to a stimulus which is normally painful' (Merskey, 1986). Primary hyperalgesia occurs at the site of injury and secondary hyperalgesia occurs in the healthy tissue that surrounds the injury. Allodynia is defined as: 'Pain due to a stimulus which does not normally provoke pain' and may be considered as tenderness (Merskey, 1986). The presence of spontaneous ongoing pain in the absence of any stimuli also serves to immobilize the structure to aid recovery. The duration of acute pain is closely related to the severity of the injury and the time course for healing.

Chronic pain is defined as 'pain lasting for long periods of time. Chronic pain commonly persists beyond the time of healing of an injury and frequently there may not be any clearly identifiable cause' (Ready and Edwards, 1992). Pain may persist for many reasons including ongoing tissue damage (nociception) as in advanced cancer, a persistent neurological condition (for example, multiple sclerosis) or a degenerating disease (for example, arthritis) (Woolf, 1994) (Figure 2.8). However, in some cases the aetiology of chronic pain is difficult to identify especially when pain persists despite the apparent healing of the injury. This may be because the nociceptive system itself may have become dysfunctional (Table 2.1).

Normal, suppressed and sensitized pain

The nociceptive system appears to operate in different states (Table 2.2) (Doubell, Mannion and Woolf, 1999). In its normal state, the nociceptive system generates transient pain sensations so that avoidance behaviour can

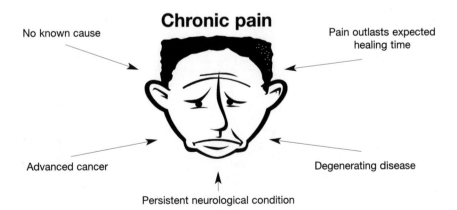

Figure 2.8 Aetiology of some chronic pains.

Table 2.2 The characteristics of normal, suppressed and sensitized pain. (Adapted from Doubell et al., 1999.)

Status of nociceptive system	Nociceptive transmission through CNS	Status of peripheral tissue	Afferent input	Sensation	Clinical correlate
Normal	Normal	Healthy	Non-noxious	No pain	Transient pain – little long-term consequence
			Noxious	Pain	
Suppressed	Diminished: reduced excitation increased inhibition	Healthy or injured	Non-noxious	No pain	Pain relief
			Noxious	Reduced pain	
Sensitized	Amplified: increased excitation reduced inhibition	Injured	Non-noxious	Allodynia (pain)	Inflammatory pain
			Noxious	Hyperalgesia (exaggerated pain)	Neuropathic pain
Reorganized	Amplified or abnormal	Healthy or injured	Non-noxious	Allodynia (pain)	Neuropathic pain
			Noxious	Hyperalgesia (exaggerated pain)	

CNS, central nervous system.

be instigated and so that we can remember to avoid the stimulus in the future. In its normal state, the nociceptive system generates pain that usually mirrors the intensity of the stimuli. In its suppressed state, the nociceptive system generates pain sensations that are lower than expected from the stimulus. This occurs in situations such as important sporting events when actions need to be completed despite the presence of noxious stimuli. Pain suppression is commonly achieved by rubbing parts of the body close to the site of injury or by mental activities like distraction and motivation. In its sensitized state, the nociceptive system generates acute pain sensations that are of greater intensity than expected such as tenderness (allodynia) and exaggerated or amplified pain (hyperalgesia). This encourages behaviours that guard the injury from additional stimuli that may hinder tissue healing.

Time course of an injury

The types of pain and changes in sensitivity of the nociceptive system can be clearly seen if you follow the time course of events that occur after a typical 'household injury' (Figure 2.9). If you hit your finger with a hammer you immediately withdraw your hand in a reflex action. This withdrawal reflex is a rapid response to remove your finger from the source of the danger and to prevent any additional accidental hammer blows. The withdrawal reflex often occurs before you experience pain. After a few seconds a sharp, intense, localized pain occurs in the finger, which is followed by a dull, aching, spreading pain. These first (fast) and second (slow) transient pain sensations result from direct activation of the nociceptive system operating in its normal state. Rubbing the body close to the injury provides some pain relief as it suppresses the nociceptive system. If appreciable tissue damage has occurred the injury becomes inflamed and is characterized by oedema, redness and soreness, with sensations of spontaneous pain, allodynia and hyperalgesia. The nociceptive system is now operating in a sensitized state. As the tissue heals with time the nociceptive system returns to its normal state and spontaneous pain, allodynia and hyperalgesia disappear. However, sometimes the nociceptive system fails to revert to its normal state and remains sensitized despite the apparent healing of tissue. In this situation the nociceptive system itself may have become dysfunctional leading to a chronic pain condition.

The physiology of nociception – normal state

The internal environment of the body is monitored by sensory receptor cells that send information to lower levels of the CNS (such as the brain

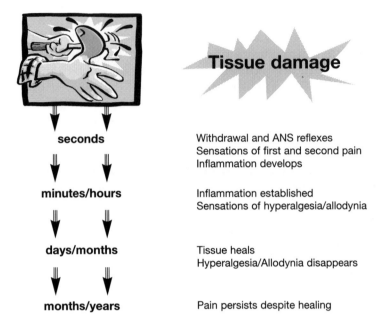

Figure 2.9 Time course of an injury. ANS, autonomic nervous system.

stem and spinal cord). Information about noxious events arriving at the CNS may generate nociceptive reflexes and/or the sensation of pain.

Nociceptive reflexes

Reflexes are fundamental to survival as they produce rapid, involuntary and predictable responses to stimuli. The nociceptive system evolved to detect stimuli that produce potential or actual tissue damage and to elicit responses that remove the noxious stimuli. This can be achieved without necessarily having to generate painful sensations.

Withdrawal (somatic) reflexes

All of us have stepped on something sharp or hot and lifted our leg in a reflex action without thinking about it and before the sensation of pain has been generated. If you had to wait for the information about the noxious stimulus to travel to the brain and for your brain to process it, generate a pain sensation and then decide and execute the most appropriate response you would probably incur a significant amount of tissue damage. The neural circuitry involved in the withdrawal reflex forms the building blocks of the nociceptive system (Figure 2.10).

Noxious, or tissue-damaging, stimuli are detected by nociceptors. These have been defined as: '[sensory] receptor(s) preferentially sensitive to a noxious stimulus or to a stimulus which would become noxious if pro-longed' (Merskey, 1986). Nociceptors are tissue-damage receptors rather than pain receptors as the brain, not the receptors, produces the ultimate sensation of pain. In battlefield analgesia, nociceptors are clearly active without a person experiencing pain (Beecher, 1955). Nociceptors convert noxious stimuli into nerve impulses in a process called transduction. The nerve impulses travel to the spinal cord along peripheral transmission pathways. The spinal cord acts as a link between the incoming information from nociceptors and the outgoing information sent along the motor neurons to skeletal muscles to generate the response. During the withdrawal reflex excitatory interneurons in the spinal cord switch on activity in the motor neurons that innervate flexor muscles so that more nerve impulses reach the neuromuscular junction generating the release of acetylcholine (Figure 2.10). Acetylcholine is a neurotransmitter that binds to and activates nicotinic receptors that are present on the post-synaptic membrane of skeletal muscle fibres and this triggers a sequence of events that leads to muscle contraction. Inhibitory interneurons in the spinal cord switch off activity in the motor neurons that innervate extensor muscles so that fewer nerve impulses reach the neuromuscular junction reducing the

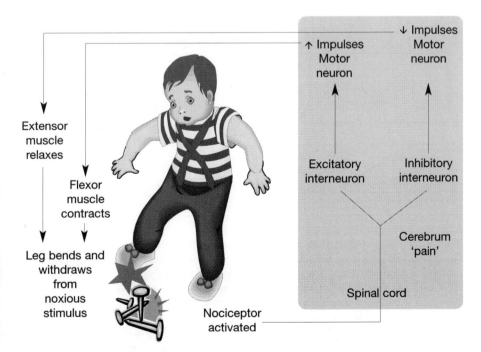

Figure 2.10 The withdrawal reflex. Arrows indicate flow of neural information.

release of acetylcholine. Therefore the extensor muscle remains relaxed. This coordination of the contraction and relaxation of opposing muscle groups is necessary to move body parts away from the noxious stimuli (Dubner and Ren, 1999).

The consequence of activity in the neural circuitry that forms the withdrawal reflex is seen in some patients who have sustained skeletal muscle contractions resulting from sustained nociceptor activity (Figure 2.11). This nociceptor-induced muscle activity is potentially damaging because it creates a positive feedback loop of contraction producing additional contraction and pain that is greater than the original stimulus (Andersson and Kokota, 1987).

Sympathetic (autonomic) reflexes

Noxious stimuli also initiate autonomic nervous system (ANS) reflexes that increase sympathetic activity, producing vasoconstriction in peripheral

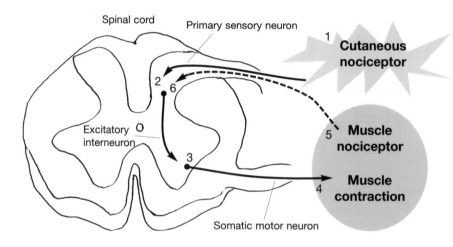

Figure 2.11 Motor reflexes contributing to pain. When cutaneous nociceptors become active (1) they send neural information to the dorsal horn of the spinal cord causing activation of interneurons (2) which release excitatory neurotransmitters (3). The resultant activity in somatic efferent neurons releases acetylcholine at the neuro-muscular junction producing a muscle contraction (4), which leads to ongoing muscle contraction and muscle spasm detected in muscle nociceptors (5). The afferent information arising from muscle nociceptors (dashed line) itself generates further muscle contraction via a positive feedback loop using excitatory interneurons and somatic motor neurons (6).

tissue leading to ischaemia (Figure 2.12). The ischaemia is detected by nociceptors, which initiate a reflex increase in sympathetic activity, additional
ischaemia and further activity in nociceptors. The sympathetically induced
ischaemia may contribute to pain in conditions such as fibromyalgia where
patients experience pain, weakness and stiffness in skeletal muscle.
Sympathetic reflexes also increase circulating levels of noradrenaline (norepinephrine) which can sensitize nociceptors and change smooth muscle
activity in other parts of the body such as the gastrointestinal tract, creating pain that is not directly linked to the original stimulus (Andersson and
Kokota, 1987).

Increased sympathetic activity also produces a stress response, sometimes
called the fight–flight–fright response, resulting in widespread physiological
changes in the body. These changes include changes in pulmonary ventilation (breathing), increased heart rate and reduced gastrointestinal motility
and bladder emptying which contribute to adverse effects such as altered
blood gas concentrations, hypertension, constipation and urinary retention
respectively (see Figure 2.1). In the short term this reflex stress response is

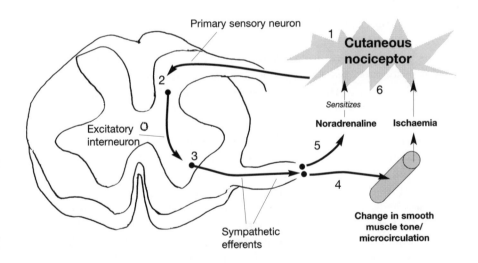

Figure 2.12 Sympathetic reflexes contributing to pain. When a cutaneous nociceptor
becomes active (1) it sends neural information to the dorsal horn of the spinal cord
(2) causing the activation of interneurons that release excitatory neurotransmitters
(3). The resultant activity in pre-ganglionic and post-ganglionic sympathetic neurons
causes vasoconstriction in peripheral tissue leading to ischaemia (4) and the release of
noradrenaline (norepinephrine) which sensitizes cutaneous nociceptors (5). The
resultant ischaemia and noradrenaline increase activity in cutaneous nociceptors (6)
and further input into the spinal cord, creating a positive feedback loop.

regulated by the release of noradrenaline from post-ganglionic efferent nerve fibres and by adrenaline (epinephrine) from the adrenal medulla. Noradrenaline and adrenaline accumulate at the site of injury and are known to sensitize cutaneous nociceptors contributing to hyperalgesia. If the stimulus persists stress hormones such as cortisol, thyroid hormones and human growth hormone are released as part of a resistance reaction to help the body fight the stressor. Cortisol breaks down fats and proteins to provide the body with additional sources of energy and it is also a potent anti-inflammatory agent. So if pain persists and the body is exposed to high concentrations of cortisol muscle wasting, suppression of the immune system and gastrointestinal tract ulceration can occur. Clearly, patients must receive appropriate pain-relieving interventions to reduce the plethora of reflex-induced physiological changes that occur as a result of nociceptor activity.

The sensation of pain

Fortunately, our behaviours are not entirely governed by reflexes. If they were we would be unable to save a child who had fallen into a fire because every time we placed our hand close to the fire it would be withdrawn in a reflex action. We have the ability to over-ride the withdrawal reflex in order to remove the child from the flames. However, our memory of previous encounters with fire makes us aware of the potential consequences of our actions because we know that placing our hands in fire is painful and that pain is associated with tissue damage. Sensations and emotions provide flexibility to the way that we can respond to stimulus by helping to drive the direction, intensity and persistence of behaviours.

We learn to avoid stimuli that produce pain because they are likely to damage our tissue. Pain sensations also create unpleasant emotions that reinforce the aversion to the stimuli. Individuals with congenital insensitivity to pain do not have physiological circuitry to detect noxious stimuli and therefore they do not learn to avoid damaging temperatures, pressures and chemicals. They often have injuries resulting from encounters with stimuli that most people avoid such as pressure sores from prolonged sitting or kneeling or loss of teeth from chewing hard objects. They often have missing digits because of accidents with hot or sharp objects. In healthy individuals the physiological circuitry to detect noxious stimuli consists of nociceptors and peripheral transmission pathways, central transmission pathways and processing by the cerebrum.

Nociceptors and peripheral transmission pathways

Nociceptors are free nerve endings that respond to high-intensity thermal and mechanical stimuli and to noxious chemicals produced by the body following injury. Peripheral transmission fibres are often described in relation to their nociceptors.

A-fibre nociceptors form small-diameter myelinated afferents (A-delta) which send action potentials into the CNS at conduction velocities above 2 ms^{-1} although they are usually in the 25 ms^{-1} range (A-delta) (Figure 2.13) (Raja et al., 1999). They respond best to extremes of hot and cold and to high intensity mechanical events producing sensations associated with 'first' or 'fast' pain. A-fibre nociceptors provide discriminative information about the noxious stimuli, such as precise location. They are often linked to 'pricking', 'sharp' and 'severe' pain. A-fibre nociceptors have been sub-classified into type 1 with a predominance of A-fibre mechanothermal nociceptors and type 2 that are less responsive to mechanical stimuli. Both types of A-fibre nociceptor are likely to be sensitive to irritant chemicals.

C-fibre nociceptors also respond to noxious thermal and mechanical events but are particularly sensitive to chemicals released during cell damage such as hydrogen ions (H$^+$), potassium ions (K$^+$), serotonin (5-HT) and bradykinin (Figure 2.13). They form small-diameter, unmyelinated afferents and have slower conduction velocities than A-fibre nociceptors (below 2 ms^{-1}, usually in the 0.5 ms^{-1} range). Information travelling in C-fibre nociceptors reaches the brain after that arising from A-fibre nociceptors and is

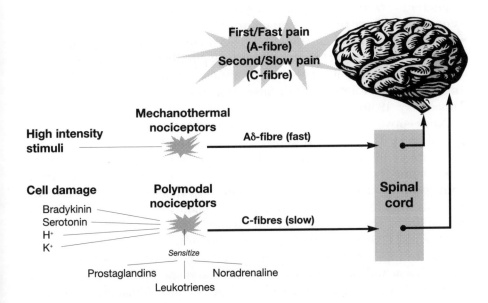

Figure 2.13 A-fibre and C-fibre nociceptors. C-fibre nociceptors are directly activated by certain substances released by cell damage and are sensitized by certain chemical byproducts of cell damage. Receptor subtypes exist for A-fibre and C-fibre nociceptors and it is likely that there is some overlap in stimuli for activation between the groups.

likely to contribute the 'second' or 'slow' pain sensations that are 'dull' and 'aching' in character.

This description of nociceptors is perilously simplistic. Many subtypes of nociceptor have been described and nomenclature can be complex. For example, nociceptors that respond to thermal, mechanical and chemical stimuli are often called polymodal nociceptors and a significant proportion of C-fibre nociceptors is likely to be polymodal. However, it is now known that many A-fibre nociceptors are also polymodal. In addition, non-nociceptive receptors are known to signal pain when the nociceptive system becomes sensitized.

Central transmission pathways

Peripheral nociceptive afferents influence activity of nociceptive transmission neurons in the spinal cord and brain stem. These central nociceptive transmission neurons project to higher brain centres such as the reticular formation, thalamus and hypothalamus (Figure 2.14). The central nociceptive transmission neurons are activated directly by peripheral afferents or indirectly by interneurons, which are themselves under the influence of peripheral and central inputs. These interneurons not only influence the activity of projection neurons but also coordinate somatic and sympathetic efferent activity involved in reflex responses. Two commonly described central nociceptive transmission neurons are nociceptive-specific (NS) neurons and wide dynamic range (WDR) neurons. These neurons form pathways which project to the thalamus (spinothalamic tracts, STTs), the brain-stem reticular formation (spinoreticular tract, SRT), and the hypothalamus and forebrain spinohypothalamic tract, SHT) (Craig and Dostrovsky, 1999).

Nociceptive-specific neurons are predominantly found in lamina I of the dorsal horn. They respond to high-intensity stimuli and transmit information rapidly in direct pathways like the spinothalamic tract from which information is sent to sensory areas of the cerebrum (for example, somatosensory cortex) to signal the intensity, quality and location of the noxious stimuli. WDR neurons are predominantly found in lamina V of the dorsal horn. They respond to non-noxious and noxious stimuli including A-fibre and C-fibre nociceptors and A-fibre 'touch' afferents, hence 'wide dynamic range'. WDR neurons form multi-synaptic pathways projecting to the reticular formation in the brain stem and the limbic system and the frontal lobes in the cerebrum. Central nociceptive transmission neurons also project to the hypothalamus via spinohypothalamic tracts to elicit sympathetic changes as described earlier.

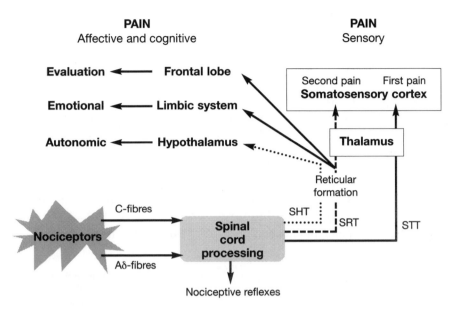

Figure 2.14 Nociceptive pathways and their relationship to sensory, affective and cognitive dimensions of pain. SHT, spinohypothalamic tract; SRT, spinoreticular tract; STT, Spinothalamic tract.

Processing of noxious information by the cerebrum

The role of the cerebrum in generating painful sensations has attracted much interest over the last decade due to improved neuroimaging techniques such as positron emission tomography (PET) and functional magnetic resonance imaging (fMRI). When healthy subjects experience experimentally induced pain a variety of brain areas becomes active in line with our understanding of the anatomy of the nociceptive system. For example, activity has been reported in the thalamus and somatosensory cortex (sensory dimensions), the cingulate gyrus and insula (affective dimensions), and the prefrontal cortex (cognitive dimensions) (Ingvar and Hsieh, 1999). Interestingly, patients with chronic pain exhibit different patterns of brain activity when compared with healthy subjects experiencing experimentally induced pain. For example, the thalamus has been found to decrease its activity in patients with chronic neuropathic pain. Clearly, there is no brain centre purely devoted to pain experience and different brain areas may become active when pain arises in different situations.

The physiology of nociception – suppressed state

Activity in the nociceptive system can be suppressed as described by the gate-control theory of pain. The 'pain gate' is opened by activity in peripheral nociceptor transmission pathways (A-fibre and C-fibre nociceptors), releasing excitatory neurotransmitter substances on to central nociceptive transmission neurons and resulting in the onward transmission of noxious information to the brain. The 'pain gate' can be closed by activity in large-diameter A-fibres that transmit non-noxious information about touch and pressure, possibly via interneurons releasing inhibitory transmitter substances such as γ-aminobutyric acid (GABA) and enkephalins (Figure 2.15). This results in inhibition of central nociceptor neurons and a reduction in the transmission of noxious information from the spinal cord to the brain. Rubbing the skin close to painful or damaged areas of the body is the simplest way to generate non-noxious A-fibre activity, hence 'rubbing the pain better'. TENS uses electrical currents to selectively activate non-noxious

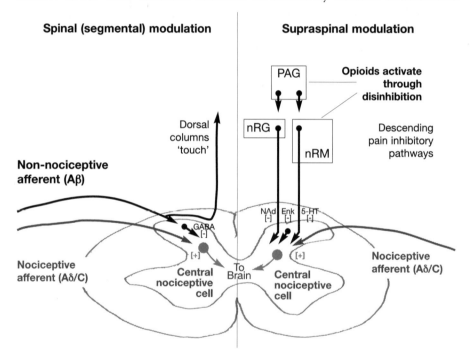

Figure 2.15 Endogenous pain suppression systems. Two main systems reduce activity in central nociceptive projection cells. Spinal modulation takes place via activity in non-noxious afferents such as Aβ 'touch' fibres, which inhibit ongoing activity in central nociceptive transmission cells through an inhibitory interneurons (–) releasing γ-aminobutyric acid (GABA). Supraspinal modulation takes place via descending pain inhibitory pathways influencing brain-stem structures like the periaqueduatal grey (PAG), nucleus raphe magnus and nucleus raphe gigantocellularis (nRG). Neurotransmitters implicated in descending pain inhibitory pathways include opioids, noradrenaline/norepinephrine (NAd), 5-hydroxytryptamine (5-HT) and enkephalin (Enk). Excitatory [+], inhibitory [–].

A-fibre without activating peripheral nociceptive transmission fibres in order to close the pain gate and produce pain relief for patients. In many respects TENS 'electrically rubs pain better'. Physiological studies demonstrate that activity of central nociceptive transmission neurons is markedly reduced during TENS (Garrison and Foreman, 1994).

The 'pain gate' can also be closed by activity in descending pain inhibitory nerve pathways that arise from supraspinal ('above spinal cord') structures. The periaqueductal grey (PAG) and the raphe nuclei (for example, nucleus raphe magnus and nucleus raphe gigantocellularis) are important brain-stem nuclei that process information in the descending pain inhibitory pathways, and these structures reduce nociceptive activity and pain when stimulated. Descending pain inhibitory pathways reduce activity in central nociceptive transmission neurons by a variety of mechanisms. They directly inhibit central nociceptive transmission neurons or indirectly inhibit central nociceptive transmission neurons through inhibitory interneurons (Figure 2.15). Presynaptic inhibition of peripheral nociceptive transmission terminals also occurs, reducing the amount of excitatory neurotransmitter released. The involvement of multiple inhibitory mechanisms implicates many transmitter substances including opioid peptides, serotonin and noradrenaline (acting on α_2-receptors) (Fields and Basbaum, 1999).

The physiology of nociception – sensitized state

Under normal physiological conditions, low-intensity mechanical stimuli are detected by mechanoreceptors and processed by the nervous system to produce non-painful mechanical sensations such as 'touch' and 'movement'. Similarly, thermal stimuli are detected by thermoreceptors to generate non-painful 'hot', 'warm' and 'cold' sensations. High-intensity, potentially damaging mechanical and thermal stimuli are detected by nociceptors and can produce painful sensations. However, if the skin is damaged due to disease or injury low-intensity stimuli may produce pain (allodynia) and high-intensity stimuli may produce severe pain, which is exaggerated in intensity (hyperalgesia). For example, applying moderate pressure to a bruise may produce pain and accidentally knocking it against an object may produce pain that is far higher than would be expected for healthy tissue. This sensitivity to stimuli helps to elicit behaviours that protect injured sites from further damage, like guarding the bruised tissue. This sensitivity to stimuli is known to occur following injury to cutaneous, visceral and muscle tissue and is due to changes in the physiology of peripheral tissue (peripheral sensitization) and central nervous system (central sensitization) (Figure 2.16).

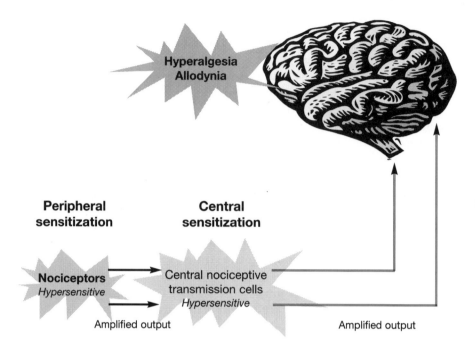

Figure 2.16 Peripheral and central sensitization.

Peripheral sensitization

When cells are damaged through injury or disease algesic (pain-producing) substances accumulate in the extracellular fluid. Some of these algesic substances directly leak out of damaged cells (Figure 2.17). Others are synthesized from non-algesic precursor chemicals that have themselves leaked out of damaged cells or have arrived in the area as a result of plasma extravasation ('outside vessel') or lymphocyte migration (Figure 2.17). In addition, nerve impulses generated by the nociceptors invade distal branches of its own free nerve endings resulting in the secretion of substance P into the surrounding tissue fluid (Figure 2.17). The chemical soup that accumulates at the site of injury produces vasodilatation, increased blood flow, increased permeability of blood vessels and plasma extravasation, resulting in symptoms of redness, heat and swelling. In addition, algesic substances activate and sensitize nociceptors, resulting in pain that tends to occur when the inflamed area is touched or moved rather than being spontaneously present in the absence of stimuli (Levine and Reichling, 1999).

C-fibre nociceptors have a fundamental role in the detection of algesic substances released as a consequence of tissue damage. Some of the substances (for example, bradykinin, 5-HT, H^+, and K^+) directly activate C-fibre nociceptors, generating action potentials that propagate to the CNS. Other substances (such as prostaglandins, leukotrienes, noradrenaline, adenosine, adenosine 5-triphosphate [ATP] and nitric oxide) sensitize nociceptors by lowering their threshold of activation so that the nociceptors begin to fire at lower intensities of stimuli. As the algesic substances begin to accumulate and diffuse into the tissue fluid they may alter the physiology of surrounding tissue. However, current evidence suggests that this does not produce any appreciable sensitization of nociceptors or contribute to secondary hyperalgesia in the healthy tissue that surrounds the injury (Raja et al., 1999).

Non-steroidal anti-inflammatory drugs (NSAIDs) such as ibuprofen and diclofenac as well as aspirin act peripherally to reduce the formation of

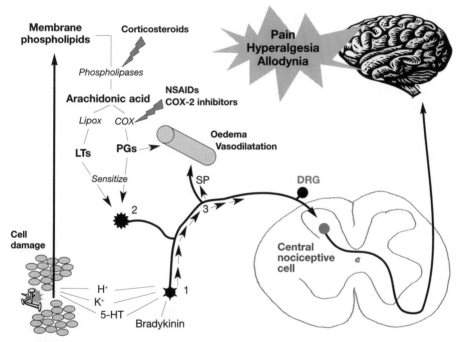

Figure 2.17 Peripheral events following cell damage. Substances released as a result of cell damage directly activate nociceptors (1). Cell damage also leads to the synthesis of leukotrienes (LTs) and prostaglandins (PGs) which act to sensitize nociceptors (2) and contribute to the inflammatory response through vasodilatation and plasma extravasation. Afferent impulses also invade the free nerve endings of the nociceptor causing the release of substance P (SP) which also causes vasodilatation and plasma extravasation (3). LT and PG synthesis is catalysed by a variety of enzymes including phospholipases, lipoxygenases (Lipox) and cyclo-oxygenases (COX) that can be inhibited by corticosteroids, NSAIDs and COX-2 inhibitors. DRG, dorsal root ganglion.

prostaglandins and are the most commonly used analgesics for the management of inflammatory pain. NSAIDs inhibit the activity of the enzyme cyclo-oxygenase (COX) which catalyses the formation of prostaglandins (PGs) from arachidonic acid at the site of tissue damage. Prostaglandins have a variety of actions throughout the body including sensitization of nociceptors. Inhibiting the activity of COX NSAIDs reduces the synthesis of PGs and therefore peripheral sensitization. COX exists in two isozymes (COX-1 and COX-2) with COX-2 being responsible for the synthesis of PGs involved in inflammation and sensitization of nociceptors. Many NSAIDs are non-selective and inhibit both isozymes, producing gastric side effects due to the presence of COX-1 in the gastric mucosa. Recently, drugs that selectively act on COX-2 have been developed in an attempt to reduce side effects and improve efficacy. These COX-2 inhibitors (such as celecoxib, etodolac, rofecoxib and meloxicam) are now used for short-term treatment of acute inflammation in joints caused by arthritis (Seibert et al., 1994).

Central sensitization

Neural information arising from the site of tissue damage enters the CNS in the dorsal horn of the spinal cord where a complex array of processing takes place leading to sensitization of central nociceptive neurons (Figure 2.18). C-fibre nociceptor input following cell damage contributes to a second pain sensation, which is known to increase in intensity over time. This has been termed 'wind-up' and is due to a decline in the threshold of excitation of central nociceptive transmission neurons with NMDA (n-methyl d-aspartate) receptors (Dickenson and Sullivan, 1987). This 'wind-up' results in central nociceptive transmission neurons amplifying their output to noxious and non-noxious inputs, resulting in hyperexcitability within the CNS and exaggerated pain sensations. The receptive fields of central nociceptive transmission neurons also expand so that they become responsive to stimuli applied to areas of tissue that do not normally activate them. Furthermore, inputs from large-diameter, non-noxious, A-beta-fibres normally associated with touch and innocuous stimuli start to activate central nociceptive transmission neurons contributing to allodynia and secondary hyperalgesia (Cousins and Power, 1999; Doubell, 1999; Raja et al., 1999).

The pharmacology of central sensitization has received much attention and is complex. The central terminals of peripheral nociceptive afferents release a variety of neurochemicals, which can be broadly divided into peptides (for example, substance P, calcitonin gene-related-peptide [CGRP], somatostatin, vasoactive intestinal polypeptide [VIP]) and amino acids (such as glutamate), although other candidate transmitters exist (such as nerve growth factor and nitric oxide) (Yaksh, 1999). These neurochemicals act on various receptors including neurokinin receptors (for example,

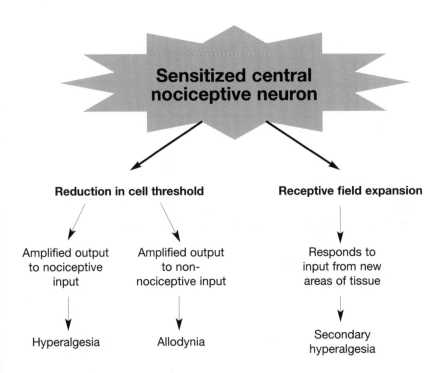

Figure 2.18 Properties of sensitized central nociceptive neurons.

substance P) and NMDA receptors (for example, glutamate). It is the action of these neurochemicals that makes central nociceptive transmission neurons hypersensitive to additional incoming noxious and non-noxious information. The NMDA receptor, which is located on the membrane of the central nociceptive projection neurons, has received much attention because of its potential role in the transition from acute to chronic pain.

NMDA receptors are activated by sustained release of glutamate and substance P from peripheral nociceptive afferent input (Figure 2.19). This causes an influx of Ca^{++} into the central nociceptive transmission neuron, which sets in motion a sequence of events that changes the neuron's excitability and structure. This results in reorganization of neuronal circuitry within the CNS (central neuroplasticity). The NMDA antagonist ketamine has been used with variable success in an attempt to prevent the onset of central sensitization for neuropathic pain, skin pain from burns and cancer pains. Pre-emptive analgesic interventions have also been used prior to surgical procedures to reduce potential long-term consequences of central sensitization associated with postoperative pain.

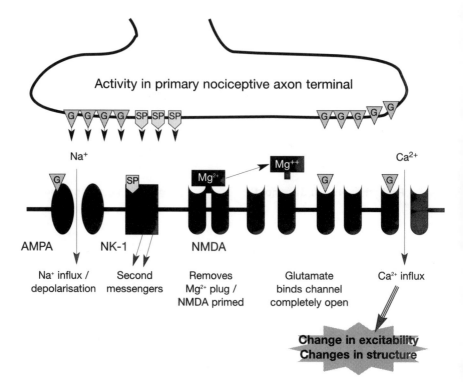

Figure 2.19 NMDA (n-methyl-d-glutamate) receptor action. A high level of afferent activity in nociceptor afferents leads to the release of glutamate (G) and substance P (SP). The neurotransmitters may be released from separate fibres or co-released from the same fibre. The NMDA receptor is primed by the removal of Mg^{2+} which takes place by concurrent activation of AMPA receptors, which depolarizes the central nociceptive neuron, and the activation of neurokinin (NK-1) receptors, which activate second messengers. Glutamate also activates the NMDA receptor to open the Ca^{2+} channel leading to long-term changes in the structural and functional abilities of the central nociceptive cell.

The physiology of damaged nerves – chronic pain state

Much of the discussion to date highlights the action of a 'healthy' nociceptive system that can change its sensitivity according to circumstance. The sensitized nociceptive system assists healing of tissue and should revert to its normal presensitized state once the tissue healing has taken place. If tissue damage persists because of ongoing degenerative disease, activity in the nociceptive system may also persist leading to chronic pain. However, sometimes the nociceptive system does not revert to its normal presensitized state despite the apparent healing of peripheral tissue, resulting in prolonged central sensitization and persistent pain. This is particularly familiar when there has been damage to nervous tissue.

Neuropathic pain

Proximal and distal nerve lesions

Pain resulting from injury to neural tissue is termed neuropathic pain and includes a range of conditions observed in the clinic such as postamputation pain in the stump, phantom limb pain, nerve entrapment, postherpetic neuralgia, trigeminal neuralgia, brachial plexus avulsions and nerve damage associated with metabolic and/or nutritional status. Neuropathic pain is characterized by pain on movement, tenderness, spontaneous dysaesthesias and spontaneous pain. Patients with neuropathic pain often describe unusual sensations such as 'shooting', 'burning' and 'electrical' coupled with mechanical and/or thermal allodynia and hyperalgesia. There are differences in the aetiology, clinical presentation and response to treatment for the variety of neuropathic pains because of the number of contributing factors (Figure 2.20) (Devor and Seltzer, 1999).

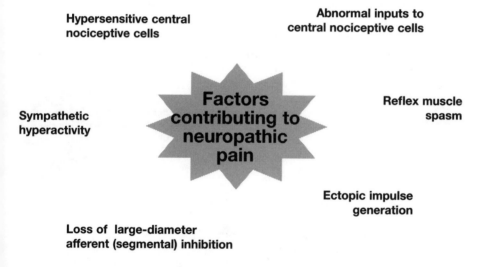

Figure 2.20 Factors contributing to neuropathic pain.

When peripheral nerves are damaged distal to the cell body, as happens in deafferentation syndromes such as limb amputations and peripheral neuropathies, the distal branches of the nerve fibre initially degenerate. A process of regeneration whereby axonal sprouts appear and attempt to re-innervate their peripheral target follows this (Figure 2.21). A clump of regenerating neuronal sprouts, termed a neuroma, forms when the axonal sprouts fail to find their target. Spontaneous nerve activity in the absence of stimuli (termed ectopic firing) may arise at the neuroma itself (primary site) and/or at the dorsal root ganglion (secondary site). This can generate pain in the absence of stimuli. Neuromas have also reduced thresholds of excitation so when pressure is applied to the injurious area excessive amounts of nerve impulses result, producing further sensitization of central nociceptive transmission neurons and persistent hyperalgesia and allodynia (Wall and Gutnick, 1974; Devor and Seltzer, 1999).

When nerves are damaged proximal to the cell body the lack of normal afferent input makes central nociceptive cells spontaneously hyperactive (Figure 2.22). This happens with brachial plexus avulsions when the spinal nerves are wrenched out of the spinal root leaving the patient with limb paralysis and insensitivity to touch but an ongoing spontaneous pain due to central sensitization.

Clearly, prolonged central sensitization appears to be a familiar contributing factor to pain following nerve damage. However, peripheral nerve lesions will also affect sensory, motor and autonomic nerve fibres. This will alter the normal balance of activity that resides within the CNS, which may also contribute to pain sensations. For example, lesions of large-diameter nerve 'touch' fibres will remove their effect to damp down activity in the central nociceptive neurons by 'gate-closing' mechanisms.

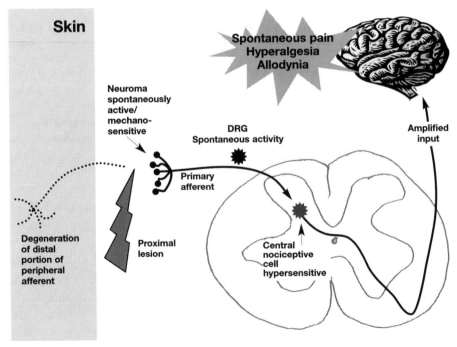

Figure 2.21 Nerve lesions proximal to the cell body of the dorsal root ganglion (DRG).

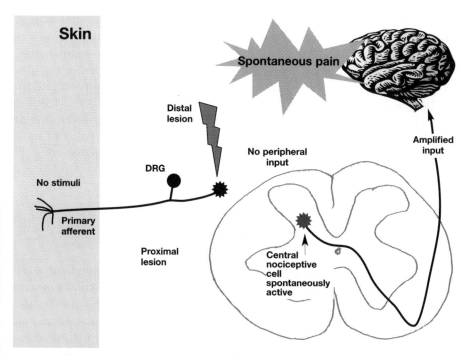

Figure 2.22 Nerve lesions distal to the cell body of the dorsal root ganglion (DRG).

Reorganization of central neuronal circuits

Nerve damage not only affects functional activity within the nervous system but also leads to structural reorganization, which can lead to irreversible peripheral and central pathophysiology. The role of reorganization of central neuronal circuits in the brain has received attention in recent years, culminating in the proposal of the neuromatrix theory of pain (Melzack, 1990). This theory attempts to explain how pain sensations appear to belong to the individual. Melzack proposed that the brain has neural circuitry that assembles somatosensory input so that somatosensations feel like our own. Melzack called this circuitry the neuromatrix and believed that it is genetically built and modified according to the patterns of nerve activity elicited by sensory input throughout life. The patterns of nerve activity, termed the neurosignature, are believed to provide a flow of sensations like pain that we recognize as belonging to ourselves.

The theory is particularly useful in explaining unusual sensations associated with deafferentation syndromes like phantom limb pain following amputation. In these situations the nervous system 'rewires' and sensations are generated in body parts that no longer exist (phantom sensations). Research has found that the loss of normal afferent input to the region of the somatosensory cortex results in reorganization of the circuitry so that areas that still have normal sensory input begin to invade areas that do not. This can generate unusual sensations such as phantom sensations including pain (Flor et al., 1995, 1998; Montoya et al., 1998). The neuromatrix theory of pain may prove very useful in developing knowledge on how nervous system damage and cortical reorganization contribute to persistent pain states.

This section emphasized the role of nerve damage in the development of neuropathic pain. However, some chronic pains, such as pains of musculoskeletal, vascular and visceral origin, do not involve neuropathy.

Deep structures contributing to pain

Deep somatic and visceral structures

Most information about the physiology of pain has been derived from studies that have focused on superficial structures such as the skin. However, many clinical pains arise from deep somatic tissue (skeletal muscle and joints) and visceral tissue (smooth muscle of the gastrointestinal, renal and vascular systems). The skin has evolved to signal encounters with noxious stimuli from the external environment and therefore generate escape behaviours coupled with a sharp and localized pain. However, nociceptors in deep somatic and visceral tissue are more likely to encounter noxious stimuli arising from damage or disease and do not respond as readily to the same stimuli as those found for cutaneous tissue. Consequently, deep somatic and visceral pain differs from cutaneous pain because it is dull, poorly localized and tends to immobolize the injured structure (Table 2.3).

Nociceptors in skeletal muscle respond to high-intensity mechanical and thermal events and to algesic agents. Skeletal muscle is very sensitive to ischaemia and generates a severe pain if the muscle contracts during the ischaemic episode. Joint nociceptors respond to extreme movements of the joint or intense pressure around the joint capsule. Joint nociceptors become sensitized during inflammation so that nociceptors begin to discharge in the absence of movement or in the presence of minor movements of the joint (Mense and Simons, 2001). It is likely that such peripheral sensitization contributes to the pains associated with the large group of chronic inflammatory joint conditions such as rheumatoid arthritis, osteoarthritis and ankylosing spondylitis.

Visceral structures such as the gastrointestinal tract, ureter and bladder are particularly sensitive to twisting, distension and chemical irritants (such as stomach acid) but are relatively insensitive to cutting, heat or pinching. It is likely that pain associated with these stimuli is subserved by A-fibre and C-fibre afferents. Pain and discomfort arising from visceral structures are one

Table 2.3 The characteristics of pain arising from superficial versus deep tissue

Characteristic	Superficial	Deep
Tissues involved	Cutaneous, mucous	Muscle including heart, smooth and skeletal; fascia, periosteum, joint and connective tissue
Intensity	Usually linked to severity of damage	Less likely to be linked to severity of damage
Quality	Sharp, pricking, stinging – definite	Dull, sore, aching – fuzzy
Location	Precise and well localized Related to site of stimulus/ source of injury and/or dermatome	Vague and poorly localized May be referred to another area of the body
Temporal aspects	More often constant than periodic	More often periodic and building to peaks of intensity than constant
Related symptoms	Autonomic symptoms occur only if tissue damage is moderate and involves deep tissue	Autonomic symptoms often present including nausea, vomiting, sweating, palpitations

Adapted from Cousins (1987).

of the most common presentations in primary care and can signal a wide range of conditions. For example, pain in the abdomen may result from appendicitis, Crohn's disease, ectopic pregnancy, biliary colic, cholecystitis, pancreatitis, gastrointestinal ulcers, carcinomas, constipation and irritable bowel syndrome, to name but a few. Pains in the chest are particularly important, as clinicians need to differentiate cardiac ischaemia from diseases of the aorta, lung or oesophagus and from disorders of somatic structures such as myofascial pain of thoracic muscles, chest injury and herpes zoster. Clearly, the aetiology and pathophysiology underlying visceral pains vary considerably and a range of different stimuli may elicit nociceptor activity (Cousins, 1987; Blendis, 1999; Procacci et al., 1999; Raja et al., 1999).

There appear to be few central nociceptive transmission neurons dedicated to visceral input and this may contribute to the poor localization of visceral pain. Deep somatic and visceral afferents are cabled in nerve bundles that primarily innervate structures like the skin or are cabled in nerve bundles with autonomic fibres like the splanchic nerve. Visceral input projects onward via spinoreticular and spinothalamic tracts as seen for cutaneous pathways and this is likely to contribute to the mechanism of referred pain.

The physiology of referred pain

Referred pain is pain that is felt at body sites that are remote from the site of tissue damage and pathology. Pathology in deep structures often produces muscle contraction, tenderness, and characteristic patterns of skin sensitivity and pain. For example, pain associated with myocardial infarction is distributed not only in the central chest beneath the sternum but also down the left arm. Pain associated with oesophageal damage is referred across the skin of the thorax and that associated with diaphragmatic damage in the shoulder. Often pain is referred to the cutaneous area innervated by the same spinal segment (dermatome) as that for the visceral structure. One theory of referred pain suggests that a single branched primary afferent arising from deep visceral and cutaneous tissue supplies the same central nociceptive transmission neuron, although evidence suggests that only a small proportion of afferent nerve cells have dual input (Figure 2.23). The convergence–projection theory of referred pain suggests that separate primary afferents arising from deep and cutaneous tissue supply the same central nociceptive transmission cell. In both instances information arising from the central nociceptive transmission cell is interpreted by the brain as coming from cutaneous afferents (Figure 2.23). This is because there are proportionately more cutaneous somatic afferent neurons converging on central nociceptive transmission neurons than there are visceral afferent neurons converging on central nociceptive transmission neurons. Hence pain sensation is more likely to be referred to cutaneous somatic structures. Nociceptive reflexes may also contribute to referred pain. Input from visceral nociceptors is known to generate a reflex muscle contraction that may be sustained and generate muscle tenderness and an additional source of nociceptive input. Hence the projection of pain arising from deep somatic and visceral structures to remote body sites, which can be a source of confusion to both clinician and patient, may be due to a combination of peripheral and central mechanisms (Fields, 1987).

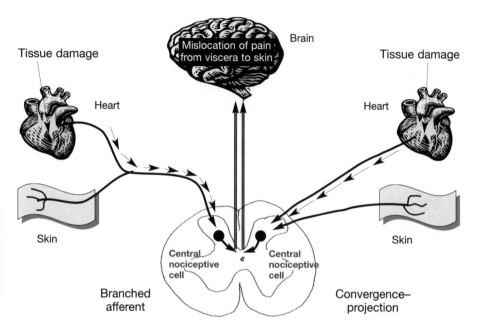

Figure 2.23 Referred pain. Branched-afferent and convergent–projection theories of referred pain result in the brain being unable to discriminate the source of the incoming noxious information (arrows) as arising from visceral structures like the heart (rather than somatic structures like the skin). This results in pain referred to somatic structures.

Conclusion

Many primary analgesic interventions in regular use today act on the outdated concept of a hard-wired 'pain pathway' (Figure 2.24). We now know that pain is not a unitary phenomenon and many factors may influence the way that we experience pain. In this chapter we have explored some of the physiological processes that contribute to the multidimensional and dynamic nature of pain sensation:

- The nociceptive system has evolved to detect stimuli that produce actual or potential tissue damage in order to elicit responses to reduce damage and aid healing.
- The nociceptive system is dynamic and its state of sensitivity can be altered.
- It converts noxious stimuli into nerve impulses in order to generate reflex responses to protect the body from (further) injury, and to yield pain sensations so that we can avoid the noxious stimuli in the future.

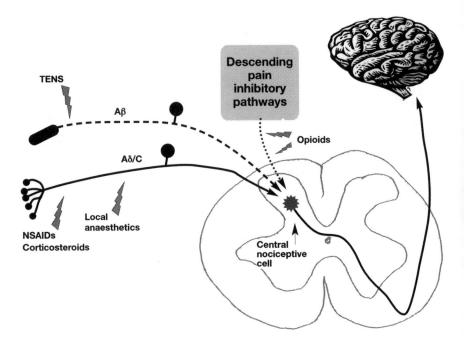

Figure 2.24 Sites of action of primary analgesic interventions.

- Nociceptive system activity can be suppressed to reduce pain sensation in circumstances where we need to escape from threatening situations.
- The nociceptive system becomes sensitive following tissue damage so that pain is amplified in order to immobilize injured body parts to promote tissue healing. This sensitization, which takes place peripherally and centrally, normally disappears when the damaged tissue heals.
- However, when there has been nerve damage the nociceptive system appears to maintain its sensitive state despite the apparent absence of ongoing tissue damage.
- This mechanism may be a significant factor in some chronic pain states and appears to be maladaptive and due to a nociceptive system that has itself become dysfunctional because of changes in its functional and structural organization in the CNS. It is therefore hardly surprising that we have such difficulty managing these chronic pain states.

References

Andersson S, Kokota T (1987) Anatomical, pathophysioloigcal and biomedical aspects of pain. In Andersson S, Bond M, Mehta M, Swerdlow M (eds) Chronic Non-cancer Pain. Lancaster: MTP Press, pp. 17–30.

Beecher H (1955) The powerful placebo. Journal of the American Medical Association 159: 1602–6.

Blendis LM (1999) Abdominal pain. In Wall PD, Melzack R (eds) Textbook of Pain. Edinburgh: Churchill Livingstone, pp. 603–19.

Cousins M (1987) Visceral disease. In Andersson S, Bond M, Mehta M, Swerdlow M. Chronic Non-cancer Pain. Lancaster: MTP Press, pp. 119–30.

Cousins M, Power I (1999) Acute and post-operative pain. In Wall PD, Melzack R (eds) Textbook of Pain. Edinburgh: Churchill Livingstone, pp. 447–92.

Craig AD, Dostrovsky JO (1999) Medulla to thalamus. In Wall PD, Melzack R (eds) Textbook of Pain. Edinburgh: Churchill Livingstone, pp. 183–214.

Devor M, Seltzer Z (1999) Pathophysiology of damaged nerves in relation to chronic pain. In Wall PD, Melzack R (eds) Textbook of Pain. Edinburgh: Churchill Livingstone, pp. 129–64.

Dickenson AH, Sullivan AF (1987) Evidence for a role of the NMDA receptor in the frequency dependent potentiation of deep rat dorsal horn nociceptive neurones following C fibre stimulation. Neuropharmacology 26: 1235–8.

Doubell TP, Mannion RJ, Woolf CJ (1999) The dorsal horn: state-dependent sensory process, plasticity and the generation of pain. In Wall PD, Melzack R (eds) Textbook of Pain. Edinburgh: Churchill Livingstone, pp. 165–82.

Dubner R, Ren K (1999) Assessing transient and persistent pain in animals. In Wall PD, Melzack R (eds) Textbook of Pain. Edinburgh: Churchill Livingstone, pp. 359–84.

Fields HL (1987) Pain. New York: McGraw-Hill.

Fields HL, Basbaum AI (1999) Central nervous system mechanisms of pain modulation. In Wall PD, Melzack R (eds) Textbook of Pain. Edinburgh: Churchill Livingstone, pp. 309–30.

Flor H, Elbert T, Knecht S et al. (1995) Phantom-limb pain as a perceptual correlate of cortical reorganization following arm amputation. Nature 375: 482–4.

Flor H, Elbert T, Mühlnickel W (1998) Cortical reorganization and phantom phenomena in congenital and traumatic upper-extremity amputees. Experimental Brain Research 119: 205–12.

Garrison DW, Foreman RD (1994) Decreased activity of spontaneous and noxiously evoked dorsal horn cells during transcutaneous electrical nerve stimulation (TENS). Pain 58: 309–15.

Gybels JM, Tasker RR (1999) Central neurosurgery. In Wall PD, Melzack R (eds) Textbook of Pain. Edinburgh: Churchill Livingstone pp. 1307–39.

Ingvar M, Hsieh JC (1999) The image of pain. In Wall PD, Melzack R (eds) Textbook of Pain. Edinburgh: Churchill Livingstone, pp. 215–33.

Levine JD, Reichling DB (1999) Peripheral mechanisms of inflammatory pain. In Wall PD, Melzack R (eds) Textbook of Pain. Edinburgh: Churchill Livingstone pp. 59–84.

Livingston WK (1943) Pain Mechanisms. New York, Macmillan.

Melzack R (1975) The McGill Pain Questionnaire: major properties and scoring methods. Pain 1: 277–99.

Melzack R (1990) Phantom limbs and the concept of a neuromatrix. Trends in Neuroscience 13: 88–92.

Melzack R, Katz J (1999) Pain measurements in persons in pain. In Wall PD, Melzack R (eds) Textbook of Pain. Edinburgh: Churchill Livingstone, pp. 409–26.

Melzack R, Wall P (1965) Pain mechanisms: a new theory. Science 150: 971–9.

Melzack R, Wall PD (1988) The Challenge of Pain. London: Penguin Books.

Mense S, Simons D (2001) Muscle Pain. Understanding its Nature, Diagnosis, and Treatment. Philadelphia: Lippincott, Williams & Wilkins.

Merskey H (1986) Classification of chronic pain. Descriptions of chronic pain syndromes and definitions of pain terms. Pain 3(suppl): S1–226.

Merskey H (1991) The definition of pain. European Journal of Psychiatry 6: 153–9.

Montoya P, Ritter K, Huse E et al. (1998) The cortical somatotopic map and phantom phenomena in subjects with congenital limb atrophy and traumatic amputees with phantom limb pain. European Journal of Neuroscience 10: 1095–102.

Noordenbos N (1959) Pain. Amsterdam: Elsvier.

Penfield W (1968) Engrams in the human brain. Mechanisms of memory. Proceedings of the Royal Society of Medicine 61: 831–40.

Procacci P, Zoppi M, Maresca M (1999) Heart, vascular and haemopathic pain. In Wall PD, Melzack R (eds) Textbook of Pain. Edinburgh: Churchill Livingstone, pp. 621–40.

Raja SN, Meyer RA, Ringkamp M et al. (1999) Peripheral neural mechanisms of nociception. In Wall PD, Melzack R (eds) Textbook of Pain. Edinburgh: Churchill Livingstone, pp. 11–58.

Ready L, Edwards WT (1992) Management of Acute Pain: A Practical Guide. Seattle: IASP Publications.

Seibert K, Zhang Y, Leahy K et al. (1994) Pharmacological and biochemical demonstration of the role of cyclooxygenase 2 in inflammation and pain. Proceedings of the National Academy of Sciences of the USA 91: 12013–7.

Tasker RR (1994) Stereotactic surgery. In Wall PD, Melzack R (eds) Textbook of Pain. Edinburgh: Churchill Livingstone, pp. 1137–57.

Treede RD, Apkarian AV, Bromm B (2000) Cortical representation of pain: functional characterization of nociceptive areas near the lateral sulcus. Pain 87: 113–19.

Wall PD, Gutnick M (1974) Properties of afferent nerve impulses originating from a neuroma. Nature 248: 740–3.

Woolf CJ (1987) Physiological, inflammatory and neuropathic pain. Advances and Technical Standards in Neurosurgery 15: 39–62.

Woolf CJ (1994) The dorsal horn: state-dependent sensory processing and the generation of pain. In Wall PD, Melzack R (eds) Textbook of Pain. Edinburgh: Churchill Livingstone, pp. 101–12.

Woolf CJ, Salter MW (2000) Neuronal plasticity: increasing the gain in pain. Science 288: 1765–9.

Yaksh T (1999) Central pharmacology of nociceptive transmission. In Wall PD, Melzack R (eds) Textbook of Pain. Edinburgh: Churchill Livingstone, pp. 253–308.

CHAPTER THREE

Living with pain through the eyes of the sufferer

KAREN MACKRODT

Aim

This chapter aims to provide the reader with an understanding of individuals suffering with chronic pain. It will pull together, from personal accounts, the complexities of chronic pain and how suffering changes the perception of those who suffer but also of those living with someone in pain.

Objectives

- To introduce the reader to the ways in which individuals view their own pain.
- To develop an understanding of how individuals in pain perceive the attitudes of the professional health team and how their attitudes towards the team have imprinted on their understanding of their pain.
- To introduce the themes generated by individuals when seeking help/cures/advice in developing an understanding of their pain.

Introduction

Pain is universal and complex and individuals react to their pain in complex ways. As professionals we can underestimate how much pain people endure on a daily basis. We may reduce their pain experience by viewing it as just a limb or painful site without looking at the far-reaching impact such pain has on them and their families.

People express themselves differently, therefore we must understand them on an individual basis. 'One cure does not cure all.' People with chronic pain appear to endure many tasks and pressures. Simple things become giant mountains to climb. Life becomes insular and the person often withdraws as the pain continues. Anyone who has ever suffered pain, whether for a few hours or a few days, will appreciate the impact that chronic pain has on individuals and their surrounding environment.

This chapter aims to encompass the thoughts and beliefs of the individual with chronic pain. Eight patients (four male, four female), known to two chronic pain services, were interviewed to develop an understanding of how they and their significant others have lived with their pain, how they dealt with it through various treatment regimens, and how they found professionals' behaviour towards them changed as the pain continued.

Nurses are directed to try to manage pain as a problem instead of attending to the person who is living the experience. Nurses tend to lead or teach about how to live with pain when it is a persistent presence. Living with chronic pain changes one's quality of day-to-day life. Numerous authors have explored the relationships among pain, suffering and quality of life (Browne, 1996; McMillan, 1996; Carson, 1998; Buchi et al., 2002; Blomqvist, 2003). Leder (1984) considered several paradoxes linked with pain. Leder claimed that pain prompts a focusing on the one sensation that is pain. At the same time, pain prompts people to look outside for relief. Relief from pain can come with movement, with things that bombard other senses (counter-stimulation) and by focusing one's attention in a different way (distraction). According to Leder, pain can restrict people from any involvement in the present yet can remind them of other times and places when pain was not present.

Living with pain

It is very difficult to imagine how you can live with a constant pain in your body. Patients in two chronic pain clinics volunteered to be interviewed for this chapter. One of the patients interviewed put it beautifully in a simple sentence: 'It isn't the pain which kills you but one that nags away at you. It is like having someone tapping away on your shoulder all the time. You can't ever brush it off.' One could infer from this statement that pain is a constant interruption.

The same person asked the question: 'When you are in pain all the time, you don't have the luxury of having days of no pain or some pain. When you are in pain all the time at what point do you tell people that you are in pain?'

To gain an insight into the lives of people in chronic pain, time was spent with individuals to gather their own story. Box 3.1 gives an overview of the interview process.

To begin with, the interview text was read several times and as open-mindedly as possible to gain a naïve understanding of the meaning of the

Box 3.1

- Eight patients known to two chronic pain clinics were interviewed.
- Patients were seen in their own homes due to the sensitive nature of the interview content. It was felt inappropriate to have them in the hospital environment as it might have detracted from the informality needed.
- One patient was interviewed in the pain clinic in a private room.
- One patient had come to the hospital when the interviewer was actually at her home so her husband, her chief carer, was interviewed instead.
- They were asked to 'Go back to the beginning and tell me your story.'
- Each interview was tape recorded and transcribed verbatim.
- All interviews averaged 2 hours.
- From the transcripts, statements were placed into contexts/themes.
- Four themes and nine subthemes were generated using Parse's human being theory (1992, 1995).
- From this the body of the chapter was born.

participants' experiences of living with pain. The text was then divided into meaning units, each consisting of a sentence, several sentences, a paragraph or several paragraphs with similar meaning in relation to the chapter aims. The meaning units were transformed through reanalysis of the context to give formulated meaning concerning the men's and women's experiences of living with chronic pain. These were then related to each other and organized into themes and subthemes (Table 3.1).

Table 3.1 Interview texts organized into themes and subthemes

Theme	Subtheme
Experiencing the body as an obstruction	Living with a reluctant body Living daily with a body in pain
Losing the 'old self'	Transcending to the past Not being in control Not being a useful person/partner/parent
Experiencing unhelpful attitudes	Not being listened to Constant battles and failures
Experiencing helpful attitudes	Gaining some control Having to nurture hope

Experiencing the body as an obstruction

The theme of experiencing the body as an obstruction consists of two sub-themes: living with a reluctant body and living daily with a body in pain. These themes relate closely to those highlighted in Paulson et al.'s (2002) study on men experiencing fibromyalgia pain.

Living with a reluctant body

All experienced some level of reluctance on the body's part to do activities because the pain stopped them from doing them. On good days one man felt a fraud. He pushed himself, especially in the garden. He'd had to give up work because of the pain. He'd stopped doing things in the garden because of the pain. He felt guilty doing the garden and not working. He said that if he could cut the grass he should be able to work. Another man carried on working after a lifting injury hurt his back. He had to drive a long distance to work. As the days went on the driving became more uncomfortable. He did all the right things – he had a hot bath, took painkillers and used hot liniments in order to be able to do the drive. Eventually he was unable to work because of the pain.

One woman was pregnant at the time and bent over and heard a 'snap' in her back. She lay on the floor and managed to get her neighbour to send for the doctor. He blamed it on the pregnancy and said it was contractions and the baby was coming. When the baby eventually came the contractions went but the back pain stayed. As the children grew the pain remained in her back. She would spend ages lying on the floor with small children around her. Her husband would get up in the morning and make sandwiches and drinks for her and the children because she couldn't stand or walk. Another man took an hour and a half to put his socks on in the morning. His wife would dress him at 4 o'clock so he could leave for work at the normal time. There were many other examples of activities that individuals wished to perform but were unable to because of their pain and disability. All found that they had the willingness in mind but inability in body to do daily tasks. They talked about not achieving or struggling with small tasks previously not even thought about.

Living daily with a body in pain

From waking to going to bed all felt the pain invaded their lives. One man described his pain as unbelievable. He described it as a 'cranking inside the head'. Every so often the pain builds up and then a bang occurs, the pain comes out and totally debilitates. All activity stops; all normal thoughts are curtailed until the pain is back under control. Severeijns et al.'s (2001) study demonstrated that chronic pain patients who catastrophize their pain experience more pain intensity, feel more disabled by their pain problem and experience more psychological distress.

Many had experienced that it was impossible at first to make plans, as they often did not know from one day to the next if they would have the energy to carry out their jobs or chores. They began to live one day at a time, sometimes minute by minute. One participant said the pain had 'chipped' away at her. She felt like 'Medusa'. Another felt she was in a cage and wished she could 'leg it' and go anywhere that didn't have any pain in it. One told of his experience of taking painkillers. He'd never taken as much as an aspirin before his back problem; now he had them for breakfast, dinner, tea and supper. Others also commented on the way that their pain altered their behaviour during the day. One woman expressed her pain to others by fidgeting from one position to the other. She found this stopped others always asking her about her pain. The meaning of living with chronic pain was uniquely presented in each description and yet all participants described their anguish and forbearance that shaped their day-to-day lives.

Losing the 'old self'

This theme consists of three subthemes: reflecting on the past, not being in control and not being a useful person/partner/parent.

In illness, the relationship to the body is changed. Instead of *being* one's body, one is confronted with *having* a body in a different way than when healthy (Paulson et al., 2002). It means losing the familiar and experiencing a sense of discontinuity with the world (Quinn, 1991). According to Corbin and Strauss (1987), chronic illness crashes into a person's life and separates the person in the present from the person in the past. In reconstructing a new timeline, the person also reconfigures his or her old self, the one that 'used to be'. This self may remain in a small or large part, but for many their physical suffering is mediated through a sense of loss (Radley, 1994).

Reflecting on the past

All the people interviewed felt cheated by the way in which the pain had changed their lives. One man was a plasterer and had been in the army and had run in marathons. When he lost the use of his legs and had to use a wheelchair he felt frustrated and angry that it had happened to him. He looked back at how he had been and what he was now. He felt humiliated at times with the pain and frustrated when it was out of control. 'You go to school, you study and you leave school. You get a job and get a house and family. That is your life. With me life stopped dead and – crash bang wallop – I had to restart my life at 40. You have to retrain your thoughts and think about your life.' Another told how her career as a nurse was 'going out of the window' and friends that she had made came to see her less and less. When she went home from hospital she felt like she had ceased to exist because she didn't see anybody, only family. All saw themselves as different from the people they once were. One man fell off a ladder, went to hospital and was told he had a crush fracture of his thoracic vertebrae and would be on traction for 6 weeks. He didn't like that idea as he was getting married within that period so he discharged himself. He now states, 40 years later, 'I find it hard to accept and it is the horrible words, "if only I had done", or '"if only I hadn't done" I wouldn't be what I am now.' (There is some self-blame here.)

All told of what they were and how much they had achieved before they had suffered with pain. They had all lived their lives to the full before the pain developed. People around them could see they were happy and full of energy. When the pain developed it wasn't only their lives that were affected but the lives of their loved ones too. Now it was a matter of getting up and surviving the day without too much distress. Pain-relieving alterations are made to habits and routines of daily life in response to the pain. One woman had her own business. So did her husband. They lost their businesses, their shop and their house through their ill health. Constant pain affects all the unseen environmental issues too. The carer highlighted the fact that his wife will not accept her limitations and where she is now: 'She thinks she can do what she did years ago. She has to set new horizons and have those that are achievable rather than the unachievable. Great advice but when you are in constant pain it isn't always easy to hear logically.' The change included remembering, keeping busy with distracting activities and retreating from others.

Not being in control

People who experience high levels of stress caused by chronic pain over a long period of time feel that nothing they do matters. They feel helpless, trapped and unable to avoid negative outcomes. As a result these people often stop striving for goals. They come to believe they have no control over their lives, and may fail to exert control over situations in which some success could be possible. They had developed what Seligman (1975) described as 'learned helplessness'. This theory demonstrated that people learn to be helpless by being in uncontrollable situations that lead to repeated failure.

One woman with back pain said that it was 'difficult' for everyone else to know what she was feeling. 'It isn't visual. Because there is nothing missing and nothing to see so your brain tells you if you see someone with one arm you know they have a problem. If you are just standing there then it isn't visible.' Many told of the frustrations felt from not being in control of their situation. To use a phrase from Chapter 1, they were experiencing themselves as people in *pain* and not *people* in pain. One told of the devastation she felt when she was told that she could no longer teach. She was due for promotion but was told to give up her job. Following this she had a disabled car sticker and couldn't get out of the car one day because of the severe pain she was experiencing. A neighbour came over and commented that 'it's all right for you to be parked in the disabled area'. She was feeling terrible and just 'let rip' at her. It made her realize that she wasn't going to cope with work and she accepted the offer of medical discharge.

According to Klinger et al. (1999) depression has been highly correlated with occupational adaptation and pain. Those individuals who adapted more activities and experienced more pain also report more feelings of depression. One man became depressed because of the constant pain he felt. Looking back he feels that he made the pain worse himself because of the constant frustration and the fact that it was always on the mind. 'It is on your mind all the time, whether your brain plays tricks with you. Other problems arise because of the state of your mind.' All told of going through stages of self-pity and 'why me?' phases. One stated that she 'played along' because she was desperate for help. She and others stated they would have done anything anyone said to them to help with the pain.

All felt the suffocating feeling of having doors shut in their faces. Time and time again, after each and every surgical procedure, they received false hopes of being pain free. All the participants had given their self-control over to the professionals at some stage and it was hard to regain that control without help from others.

Not being a useful person/partner/parent

All have found it difficult to come to terms with a less active life. None of the eight participants was working. Adjustments include spending more time at home, seeking assistance for instrumental activities of daily living such as shopping and laundry, decreasing participation in activities such as sports and social activities, and using rest during an activity in order to complete it (Henriksson et al., 1992).

The men felt useless because their role had changed within the household. Their wives were now the breadwinners. Self-esteem shifts to a negative position. The women in the group felt they were unable to do the household chores and so felt guilty in a different way because it was hard even to prepare evening meals at times because of the pain. One told of hating herself. She said 'I didn't want anyone to know how much pain I was in. I thought I had become a pain in the bum to other people. People don't want to know how much pain you really are in, so you lie to them, you hide the truth.' One woman felt she had a long way to go before she was ready for society. Throughout her twenties and thirties she had been in pain. She had lost the knack of talking socially to people. She hadn't experienced going to the pub and meeting members of the opposite sex because she had either been in hospital or at home in bed with pain.

Partners' behaviour towards them shifted too. One told of her husband becoming too protective. 'It came to the point when I dropped something he would pick it up. If I went down on my knees he would already be there before I had got down.' Another told of the reality of having to have a 'false retirement' before actually being at the age for retirement. He felt he was under pressure to go back to work even though it was a struggle. The husband of one woman felt that there had been a gradual shift in his responsibilities within the home. He found himself doing more and more of the daily routines. One man said 'I feel stupid that I do not feel like a man anymore. She's carrying three bags of shopping and I am carrying none. I wonder what she is thinking. It is degrading.'

Relationships with spouses faltered. One told: 'My relationship with my husband was very distant. My whole day was in pain, going to bed, getting up and then going back to bed. Being intimate was totally out of the question. I couldn't stand anybody near me because of the actual physical part of all that. I didn't want to do anything, not that I didn't want to, I just couldn't.'

Another told of the fact that he hadn't had a sexual relationship with his wife for over 10 years. 'I tell her I love her every day and I am always giving her cuddles and kisses. The only thing is she used to give me cuddles and squeeze me and I would lock up. So now she doesn't do that. That side of it has gone from her.' The carer stated there are many times that his wife is in pain and she sleeps a lot due to the medication, but there is no spontaneity. 'It certainly has been lost, but you just adjust to things.' One told of the fact that when she had gone out with men on dates they couldn't cope with the fact that she had a pump implanted into her abdomen. They would shy away once they found out. She believes that to have a successful relationship 'the person has to accept you for what and who you are, gadgets and all'. She felt it could be easier to continue relationships if they were already established, well before the pain problem occurs.

One man found that his twin sons were deeply affected at first. His youngest was affected the most. He said: 'At one time his dad would coach football, his dad went to work 7 days a week, his dad brought the money in, then all of a sudden there is dad unable to do anything much.' When the boys wanted new football boots he was unable to buy them so they both went out and found a little job to save up for them. The man knew that if he had still been earning they wouldn't have thought of doing anything like that. His pain had made them grow up too quickly.

Another asked her grown-up children whether they had seen her miserable all the time they were growing up without her joining in. They said no. They just accepted it as that was their life. 'We went out together and dad "did" and I sat on the side clapping and laughed, which was the way they saw it.' Another mother also felt saddened that her pain had made her children lose their childhood. She does see the positive side and feels they are very independent and confident. However, the downside of this is that she feels that she has to hide her pain from them and try to manage more than she really can to let them live their lives.

All found that when the pain is bad they become isolated in some respect with the pain. One explained that she hadn't lost her circle of friends of five or six good ones, just the hangers on. Due to not being able to work others found they missed their work colleagues and, slowly, through time, even these dwindled to only a few. Hospitals became their social life at one point or another.

Experiencing unhelpful attitudes

This theme consists of two subthemes: not being listened to and constant battles and failures.

Not being listened to

Not only did professionals fail to listen to the interviewees but members of their families and friends behaved in the same way. Madjar (1997) highlighted that pain can create a gulf between those who are in pain and those who are not. One said of his friends: 'The friends don't understand it. I ask them to trust my judgement. They don't think I can trust myself; they are even taking that away from me.' The same man stated that, one evening, his friend asked him to go to the pub. His wife asked: 'Will you be all right?' He thought: 'Why can't she leave me alone?' Many felt that they had to live their lives so they didn't upset anyone even though it caused them mental anguish to do so. Many felt that others were being overprotective when, in fact, they were smothering them with their kindness.

At the beginning many believed in what the medics told them without questioning their ability or the rate of success. One recounted that she was so naïve or desperate and that she just 'swallowed what they said'. She hadn't asked any questions about the surgery. She says: 'I remember these wonderful words ringing in my ears – you will be all right now, get on with your life, the only thing is you will never be able to ride a bike again.' Two years later she needed another operation. Again she was told that it would change her life. On the face of it she says 'I then realized the operation hadn't been the solution; on a practical level it hadn't solved anything and equally on a psychological level my hopes had been dashed again.'

Others told of being given false expectations by the surgeons that they would return to work with minimal problems. Many felt that they hadn't been given honest expectations and that the surgery would give back their life without pain. Some were given statistics to work with on how much pain relief would be gained; others were given timescales to return to work. Too often the 'caring' professionals criticized what they were doing or what they were not doing. One explained that she had seen a surgeon who hadn't a clue as to what she was feeling. He had told her that it was all in her head and there wasn't anything wrong with her because the X-rays did not show up any physical problem. She felt that he believed she was 'making it up' and the pain wasn't real.

It wasn't just the medics who expressed unhelpful attitudes towards them. One told of a physiotherapist at a rehabilitation centre who acted as if she was related to an 'SS officer'. She couldn't get down to the floor without the assistance of a chair during an exercise programme. The physiotherapist took the chair away and left her stranded for 6 hours until someone came to look for her. She was cold, hungry, desperate, exhausted and in terrific pain. This was not helpful behaviour from the professional. It left this person distraught and in too much pain to continue with the programme. She lost the trust in the professionals supposedly 'caring' for her. She didn't complain because she felt she had to play the game. Where would she go if she were discharged?

The same person found that she would inform doctors and nurses about her limitations but they appeared not to believe her. She stated they would sweep these to one side and expect her to work within their set limitations, which were unsuitable for her, and that she felt they then branded her as 'not trying'. One expressed great sadness that following a major operation she was left screaming in pain and was told to be quiet, ending up with a pulmonary embolus. She says: 'It frightened me, it really frightened me and I found a change in the nurses' attitudes. I was frightened of the nurses in case I made too much fuss.' Some nurses had compassion and others didn't. A number of nursing studies have highlighted the paradox that nursing requires nurses' participation in acts that can inflict pain and cause suffering to other human beings (Madjar, 1999; Nagy, 1999; Allcock and Standen, 2001). The participants didn't expand on their concept of the 'uncaring' nursing and medical staff they experienced but those who experienced this were hurt by the way they had been treated.

Many also expressed anguish at some of the nurses' attitudes to them while recovering from surgery. One being an ex-nurse herself said: 'The nurses don't like it if you are a nurse. I was told that because I was an orthopaedic nurse I would be able to quote all the right symptoms for the problem. In the end I asked my GP to stop putting down that I was a nurse. He thought he was being helpful, but he wasn't!' Blomqvist (2003) demonstrated that problematic, demanding or unpopular patients are considered to be uncooperative or to be coping less well and lacking visible indicators of pain.

Constant battles/failures

At the stage when these people were interviewed they had all gone through many procedures and investigations by the medical profession and many changes in their lifestyles. Many battles were against the professionals who were aiming to get them better. Lack of communication and honesty was a large theme and everyone experienced it. They were all at some point 'playing the game' to gain results with their pain at each medical hurdle. Madjar (1999) points out that carers must not doubt the reality of a person's pain but should acknowledge its existence.

Another says:

> I found the medical profession gave me an attitude over time. Through getting different diagnoses and because you can't be yourself because the pain is there all the time, and your aim is to get it sorted. It doesn't give you any room to look at different things in different ways. It is the professional's attitude that reflects on the patient. It can put doubts in your own mind that make you think that you are not in as much pain as you think you are. There were times when I didn't feel a person just the L4/5 person coming through the door and nothing else.

Hall et al.'s (1999) study demonstrated that the physician's job is to detect morbidity. Physicians have a low threshold for 'seeing' signs of emotional distress. They may also make assumptions about the distress and discontent experienced by those with chronic illness.

The husband of one woman said: 'We have tried everything to get rid of the pain. She has tried Reiki and seems to get some relief from it but it only sends her to sleep for the rest of the day. She has tried physiotherapy, massage but they all have limited effect.' Others became caught in the trap of taking more and more medication to try to reduce the pain.

One explained that she had been referred to a residential pain-management programme to improve the way she dealt with the pain. It uses a cognitive–behavioural approach. When she went up to the assessment, someone said 'you have caused all this pain by having six operations, and by the way, you are now a drug addict'. He offered her no assistance in dealing with these statements. A week later she received a letter saying if she had problems with stairs she could not come on the programme. She didn't go, but felt they wanted fit, well people for the programme.

One man now has a spinal cord stimulator in place to help with his pain (see Chapter 6 for an explanation). He underwent intensive assessment (psychological and physical) to determine whether this would be an appropriate treatment for him. He perceived that it could take 70% of his pain away. He recounted that he would have done it even if they had said that it would provide 7% relief. However, professionals working in chronic pain clinics tend to suggest that they could provide a maximum of 50% relief and anything over this is a bonus. He now says of the device 'the body gets used to it quicker than it does to drugs. I can put it on and immediately the pain goes away. The second it is switched off the pain comes back. If I have the stim on I can't move my head at all. The simplest movements can increase the intensity to unbearable mode. It normally sits on the table unattached.'

Experiencing helpful attitudes

Gaining some control

Having a chronic illness is extremely stressful. There are a number of reasons why believing that you have personal control can affect the amount of distress experienced in the face of such stress. Perceiving control may influence the predictability of outcomes. Perceiving that you are in control of the situation can set an upper limit to how bad the outcome will be. It often makes you feel better emotionally (Wallston, 1993).

Many started to shift their locus of control from believing others had the power to help them to having a greater internal locus where they started to believe in themselves again. One of the greatest changes occurred for some following attendance on pain-management programmes. One expressed it as the 'road to Damascus'. All the people on the programme were saying the same things as her. She found she could talk openly about the pain in a relaxed way. One woman felt that when she attended the chronic pain clinic: 'There was a shift that happened. Not straight away, but there was a definite shift with my thought processes and with my self-worth. If I can get back some control, try to do something positive and find myself again I can start to live again.'

Another found that following the procedure to put an implantable pump for delivering morphine into her system made a huge difference to her life. She says:

> Once I had the pump working, I felt for the first time in years awake. I would read the papers and watch the news but I wouldn't take anything in when I was taking the morphine orally. Now I am so alert I realize now what I have

been missing all these years. It was obvious that I had turned into a walking zombie. When I became awake I was seeing things for the first time. Family has noticed a difference in me; I no longer have hollow eyes. It was amazing to get up one morning and feel awake. I couldn't get used to it at first but it is so nice. I hadn't realized what I had become.

Another said:

Through using relaxation techniques I can now use it when I am hurting bad. I can separate myself, not completely so it doesn't hurt but I can distance myself. Just being able to accept it and being more objective. 'Do I have to do it?' 'No, but I don't need to avoid it completely.' I have stopped saying sorry to everyone for what I am not achieving. Now it doesn't worry me.

Participants also commented that the activities they continued to do were important, and that activities that they no longer did were less important. Therefore they had adapted how they did activities that were most important.

Others have developed their hobbies more to enable them to achieve things. One woman has become the editor of a charity newsletter while pursuing other things in her own time. Pacing becomes paramount in achieving things on a daily basis. Through pacing many were taking holidays and visiting friends again. They have learnt to develop a strategy for themselves, which works for them. Through this they have learnt to be able to 'do things again'. They had learned to alter their value systems to maintain their quality of life, for example, dropping activities that are no longer feasible and replacing them with other activities (Rejeski, 1996).

Lazarus and Folkman (1984) consider coping to be a process that changes over time and across situations. So by changing the situation or changing their feelings about it they developed more helpful coping strategies.

Having to nurture hope

Hope can be defined as 'the feeling that what is wanted can be had or that events will turn out well'. Hope is a complex human experience. It is a mixture of feelings that centre on the belief that there are solutions to human problems and needs (Lange, 1978).

Despite being pessimistic about ever being without pain in the future, all of those interviewed retained various wishes and goals in life. They had given up hope of living life without pain and had accepted that there would always be some level of pain in their lives. By believing this and striving to get the most from the situation they were living in, they had developed hope that they would get the most from what they had.

Dale Genova-Strickland (1997) expressed the experiences she had living with chronic pain. She says of the theory behind *On Death and Dying* by

Kübler-Ross (1969): 'Of the stages you go through when you learn you are terminally ill and faced with the reality that you are going to die. First, you have denial; then bargaining; then anger; then acceptance. Chronic pain is much the same. Chronic pain in its own right is terminal.' Does this suggest that pain may not totally go away until death? She says:

> Life changes because of the pain, yet you refuse to believe this has happened. That is the denial. Then comes the bargaining. No bargains can be made. Then, the anger. Angry with everyone for not realizing I hurt. Angry because I was suffering and my life was changing before me in every direction. Anger because doctors, lawyers and everyone questioned me, wanting to know. The anger only leads to more. The acceptance is when I have accepted this life with pain. It has taken five years for this acceptance to take hold. It hasn't changed the pain, it has only allowed me to laugh again.

These words from a person suffering like the eight people interviewed identifies clearly what their transition has been like. You can see that they have now attained some level of acceptance. A poem by a chronic pain sufferer of many years sums up what her feelings and thoughts about her constant pain are.

A poem by a chronic pain sufferer (June Pears)

Pain is something you cannot see, a silent partner, there
constantly.
Each morning you wake up, you hope and pray the pain won't
be as bad today.
You try to be cheerful, and carry on, hoping tomorrow the pain
will be gone.
People say 'you look well', you don't let on your days are hell.
You try to come to terms with what you have got, but peace
within, you definitely have not.
The days go by, the tears often fall, the road is long, the
mountain tall.
But day-by-day, you try your best, but life's a bitch, you've lost
your zest.
That 'get up and go', enjoy life to the full when you're in pain,
it isn't a life at all.
Miracles happen, so they say, I just hope one comes my way.
To wake up in the morning free from pain my life would be
worth living again.
To plan a future, to laugh and smile, to find peace, just for
a while.
You can't see the pain, or feel the mental stress the way you
feel, you're a total mess. But somehow your inner strength sees
you through, you hope and pray life will be kinder to you.

All the participants had started to accept, and some had gone further into accepting, that they should live their lives as best they could but all had a place in their minds that asked for a miracle to happen.

Comprehensive understanding

A life full of pain implies constant pain and the inability to lead a 'normal life'. A healthy body is taken for granted until it is no longer functioning normally. In order to lead as normal a life as possible all the sufferers had to search for relief of pain and nurtured hope despite treatment failings. Pain is more likely to cause suffering when it is out of control, its intensity is overwhelming, its source is unknown, its meaning is very serious and it shows no signs of ending.

Figure 3.1 is a pictorial representation of illness. It emphasizes the dimensions of illness and can clearly identify the themes and subthemes

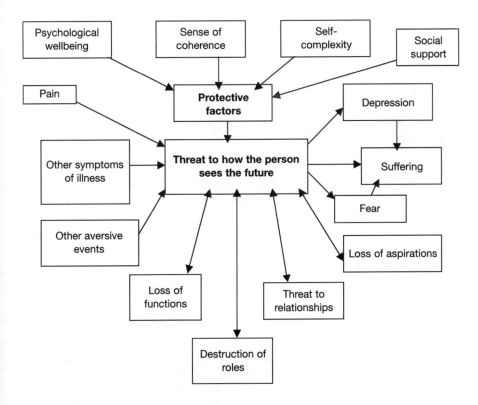

Figure 3.1 Pictorial representation of illness. (Courtesy of Tom Sensky Department of Psychological Medicine, Imperial College London, West Middlesex University Hospital.)

that the eight chronic pain participants experienced. All had varying degrees of loss of their older self and many had developed their own ways of dealing with the pain and the situation they were now in. It was interesting to hear how they had all emerged with different viewpoints and the losses at this stage in their lives were not as prominent as previously.

Conclusion

Enhanced understanding of the experience of living with chronic pain prepares nurses and health professionals to be more open to discover how individuals live in enduring discomfort. As the poem reminds us, we cannot ever truly understand another person's pain experience. Health professionals have a responsibility to listen to people if they want to speak about their pain and to respect those who do not wish to tell.

Nurses have a responsibility to learn how people want and prefer to use their medication and other therapies. Carson (1998) feels that nurses should strive to attain specific outcomes:

- all patients should have the opportunity to discuss personal concerns about pain and comfort;
- care plans should flow from the patient/family perspective of concerns and desires;
- every concern about pain should be addressed and evaluated by the patient/family.

People who live with pain learn the intricate ways in which things help and hinder, and they know how much relief they want and when it might be best to try a different strategy. Nurses and other professionals have a role, which is listening, providing comfort and acting when requested. This may be a more helpful approach to these people than gaining large amounts of information via a lengthy assessment, which can hinder nurses and professionals from truly understanding lived experiences of pain.

References

Allcock N, Staunden P (2001) Student nurses' experiences of caring for patients in pain. International Journal of Nursing Studies 38: 287–95.

Blomqvist K (2003) Older people in persistent pain: nursing and paramedical staff perceptions and pain management. Journal of Advanced Nursing 41: 575–84.

Browne R (1996) Accepting the challenges of pain management. British Journal of Nursing 5: 552–5.

Buchi S, Buddeberg C, Klaghofer R et al. (2002) Preliminary validation of PRIM (Pictorial Representation of Illness and Self Measure) – a brief method to assess suffering Psychotherapy and Psychosomatics 71: 333–41.

Carson G, Mitchell GJ (1998) The experiences of living with persistent pain. Journal of Advanced Nursing 28: 1242–8.

Corbin J, Strauss AL (1987) Accompaniments of chronic illness: changes to the body, self, biography, and biological time. Research in the Sociology of Health Care 6: 249–81.

Genova-Strickland DI (1997) Living with chronic pain. Clinical Journal of Pain 13: 178–9.

Henriksson C, Gundmark I, Bengtsson AEK (1992) Living with fibromyalgia: consequences for everyday life. Clinical Journal of Pain 8: 138-44.

Klinger L, Spaulding SJ, Polatajko HJ et al. (1999) Chronic pain in the elderly: Occupational adaptation as a means of coping with osteoarthritis of the hip and/or knee. Clinical Journal of Pain 15: 275–83.

Kübler-Ross E (1969) On Death and Dying. New York: Macmillan.

Lange S (1978) Hope. In Carlson C, Blackwell B (eds) Behavioral Concepts and Nursing Interventions. Philadelphia: JB Lippincott, pp. 171–90.

Lazarus RS, Folkman S (1984) Stress, Appraisal, and Coping. New York: Springer.

Leder D (1984) Toward a phenomenology of pain. Review of Existential Psychology and Psychiatry XIX(2–3): 256–65.

McMillan SC (1996) Pain and pain relief experienced by hospice patients with cancer. Cancer Nursing 19: 298–307.

Madjar I (1997) The body in health, illness, and pain. In Lawler J (ed.) The Body in Nursing. Melbourne, Australia, Churchill Livingstone, pp. 53–73.

Madjar I (1999) On inflicting and relieving pain. In Madjar I, Walton JA (eds) Nursing and the Experience of Illness. London: Routledge.

Nagy S (1999) Strategies used by burns nurses to cope with the infliction of pain on patients. Journal of Advanced Nursing 29: 1427–33.

Parse RR (1992) Human Being: Parse's theory of nursing. Nursing Science Quarterly 5(1): 35–42.

Parse RR (1995) Illustrations: the human being theory. In Practice and Research. New York: National League for Nursing Press.

Paulson M, Danielson E, Söderberg S (2002) Struggling for a tolerable existence: the meaning of men's lived experiences of living with pain of fibromyalgia type. Qualitative Health Research 12: 238–49.

Quinn A (1991) A theoretical model of the perimenopausal process. Journal of Nurse-Midwifery 36: 25–9.

Radley A (1994) Making Sense of Illness: The Social Psychology of Health and Disease. London: Sage, pp. 146–8.

Seligman MEP (1975) Helplessness: On Depression Development and Death. San Francisco, CA: Freeman.

Severeijns RM, Vlaeyen JWS, Van de Hout MA, Weber WEJ (2001) Pain catastrophizing predicts pain intensity, disability, and psychological distress independent of the level of physical impairment. Clinical Journal of Pain 17: 165–72.

Wallston KA (1993) Psychological control and its impact in the management of rheumatological disorders. Psychological Aspects of Rheumatic Disease 7: 281–95.

CHAPTER FOUR

Appraising pain

CAROLYN MACKINTOSH

Aim

To present an overview of the key issues that affect the appraisal of pain and to indicate how these issues can affect subsequent clinical practice.

Objectives

By the end of the chapter the reader will:

- be able to recognize the range of issues that affect the appraisal of pain;
- be able to identify the complex interrelatedness of these issues for the individual experiencing pain;
- be able to identify how these issues affect the clinical appraisal of pain;
- be aware of the skills necessary to ensure that optimum appraisal of pain can occur.

Introduction

The accurate appraisal of pain requires a creative, holistic assessment of the individual experiencing pain. This chapter identifies some of the issues that contribute towards this appraisal: the nature of pain itself, the complexity of individual variations in the experience, the ability of healthcare professionals and pain sufferers to recognize and communicate effectively the pain experience and, finally, the place of assessment as a method of attempting to overcome many of these issues.

Pain is regarded in this chapter as a consistent phenomenon, and although differences exist between the different types of commonly occurring pain (acute pain, chronic pain, malignant pain) these do not detract from the centrality of key factors in the appraisal of pain that are common throughout all its occurrences.

This chapter aims to increase awareness of these key factors and their impact on the appraisal of pain, as well as offering an insight into how assessment may offer a mechanism to improve the appraisal and subsequent management of pain for sufferers and healthcare workers.

The nature of pain

Pain is an elusive phenomenon that contains not only physiological but many humanistic and emotional qualities which ensure that the appraisal of pain is a difficult and complex task. It is the emotional and human nature of the pain phenomenon that is perhaps the most difficult concept for healthcare professionals in the present day to recognize and understand. This is clearly indicated in the rather dry definition of pain first offered by the International Association for the Study of Pain (IASP) in 1979 and now regarded as standard: 'an unpleasant sensory and emotional experience associated with actual or potential damage or described in terms of such damage' (IASP, 1979: 249).

Subsequent definitions remain equally elusive and unsatisfactory offering limited deconstructions, whether made from a personal or professional perspective, as if the intangibility of the actual pain phenomenon forms a complex barrier preventing understanding. This is no different in chronic pain, which is simply defined as 'pain that persists past the time of normal healing' (Strong, 1999: 13).

Many of the differences between chronic and acute pain are largely attributed to this longevity, exacerbating many of the issues that occur in all painful experiences, but also as a direct consequence of its persistence, giving rise to its own unique problems. These differences are summarized in Table 4.1.

However, the nature of this pain remains equally elusive and ill defined. As Degenaar (1979: 303) concludes in his argument on the nature of pain, the perspective from which the pain is viewed is perhaps the most important factor: 'neurologists speak in terms of nerve impulses, psychologists in terms of emotional qualities, philosophers in terms of sensations, feeling, suffering and meaning, and theologians in terms of guilt and punishment.'

If the nature of pain remains elusive, attempts to appraise it are automatically compromised by this inability to comprehend or define the actual phenomena. Consequently, the appraisal of pain must always be regarded as a limited and inexact skill. This does not mean that appraisal

Table 4.1 Differences between acute and chronic pain

Acute pain	Chronic pain
• Pain is a symptom	• Pain is a disease
• Well-defined onset and likely duration	• Ill-defined onset
• Identifiable pathology	• Pathology often unidentifiable
• Objective clinical signs	• Absent or adapted pathology
• Response to tissue damage	• Peripheral central changes in somato-sensory cortex
• Biological function	• Unknown biological function
• Often relieved by treatment	• Does not respond to treatment
• Associated with anxiety	• Associated with depression
• Works well with the biomedical model	• Does not work well with the medical model
• Involves the individual	• Involves the family, social network and lifestyle

Adapted from Wittink and Michel (1997).

should not be attempted but, instead, appraisal must be placed firmly within the context of this inexactitude. Appraisal of pain may never be exact, but skilled appraisal can provide a good approximation of the individual's experience and act as a firm foundation for subsequent management and treatment.

Individual variations in the pain experience

A range of factors has been accredited with determining, to a greater or lesser degree, responsibility for many of the individual variances in reported pain. Most frequently identified factors include:

- age;
- gender;
- psychological factors – personality type, anxiety, depression, prior experience and culture.

These may affect people with chronic pain in exactly the same way as all pain sufferers.

Age

There have been a number of long-standing suggestions that age influences how pain is perceived, with particular reference to the young and the elderly (Mather and Mackie, 1983; Melzack et al., 1987; Short et al., 1990; Briggs, 2003). This affects not only the sufferer of the pain but also the carer for that person. Donovon et al. (1987) reported that dissatisfaction with pain relief is higher in younger patients and this is tentatively supported by the work of Burns et al. (1989), who found that analgesic requirements of 100 patients using PCA (patient-controlled analgesia) decreased with increasing age. Where individuals are not in control of their own pain control similar findings have also been reported. Lay et al. (1996) found that the amount of prescribed and administered opioid given to 80 cardiac surgery patients decreased in patients aged 65+ and that this difference became greater as postoperative days passed.

None of these findings is conclusive and the impact of age if any remains unclear. McCaffery (1983) suggests that these differences may indicate that individuals merely express their pain differently, either as a result of age, or as result of the social norms of their own generation.

Gender

The genders of both the sufferer and the carer have also been reported as a key factor in determining individual variance; however, this is inconclusive, with Cohen (1980) and Burns et al. (1989) reporting higher levels of analgesic consumption by men, and Feine et al. (1991) also reporting, in an experimental rather than a clinical study, that gender-based sensory differences do exist. Taenzer et al. (1986), Bush et al. (1993) and Mackintosh and Bowles (1997) reported no differences in reported levels of pain between the genders in clinical subjects.

Although many healthcare professionals may cite anecdotal evidence to support gender differences in the pain experience, it appears likely that no such differences exist beyond the normal variations for each individual regardless of sex.

Psychological factors – personality types

Gender and age-related differences in individual pain perception remain inconclusive but psychological factors may have greater effect. The commonest factors so far indicated are: levels of introversion and extraversion, coping styles, anxiety traits and depression.

Taezner et al. (1986) found that extraverted patients reported more pain and consequently received more analgesics. However, in a partial replication of this study, Weisenberg and Caspi (1989) found extraversion had no significant effect on reported pain ratings or pain behaviour. The related but dissimilar issue of verbalization may cause this effect, with Hamers et al. (1996) highlighting higher levels of pain reporting by more verbal patients, as well as higher levels of recognition of pain by staff from more verbal patients.

How the individual copes with pain can also have a significant effect. Copp (1974, 1985) identified a model of pain coping styles with five different approaches:

1. type 1: pain is powerful and the coper is a passive victim;
2. type 2: the pain is invading (invader) and the coper is the combatant;
3. type 3: the pain is the reality and the coper is responsive to it;
4. type 4: the pain is cunning and the coper is reactive to it;
5. type 5: the pain is demanding and the coper is interactive with it.

Copp used this model to develop an instrument called the Pain Coping Style Inventory, which has been extensively used in work with people experiencing pain of a chronic nature (Umlauf et al., 1986; Crow et al., 1996). This work indicates that people with positive coping styles (for example, types 2 and 3) are much more likely to find ways of coping with a painful experience than people with a more negative or passive coping style (for example, types 1 and 4), who may experience higher degrees of difficulty in coping with similar amounts of pain resulting in higher levels of pain verbalization, as well as higher levels of anxiety.

Anxiety

Anxiety has also been identified as a strong indicator of individual variations in pain, with higher levels of anxiety resulting in higher reported levels of pain. Hayward (1975) was an early exponent of this link and suggested that, if giving information reduces anxiety, then postoperative pain can also be reduced. These findings are implied in the earlier work of Chambers and Price (1967) and confirmed by Taezner et al. (1986), who found that higher levels of trait anxiety and neuroticism increased pain perception, and these were the two most important factors in predicting pain responses. However, immediate preoperative anxiety (state anxiety) was not a significant factor. This is contrary to the findings of Thomas et al. (1995) who found state anxiety to be a significant predictor of postoperative pain and individuals with high levels of state anxiety gained the greatest benefit from using PCA.

It is apparent from these studies that anxiety in both forms (state and trait) is clearly linked to higher levels of reported pain, and that reductions in anxiety can also result in reductions in reported pain levels. This is of particular importance in chronic pain where the lack of identifiable pathology often leads to increased anxiety (and suspicion) about the likely underlying cause of the pain.

Depression

Depression is closely linked to trait anxiety. Taezner et al. (1986) found that depression measured the night before surgery was a more significant indicator of postoperative pain than anxiety. Depression is also closely linked to chronic pain, and is frequently appraised alongside the actual reported pain, and may contribute as many difficulties to the chronic pain sufferer as the pain itself. Levels of reported depression among chronic pain sufferers are high with a well-established interrelationship (Haley et al., 1985; Sanders et al., 1992).

Prior experience/knowledge

The individual's prior experience and expectations of pain have also been regarded as a key factor in determining individual variance (Cohen, 1980; Walmsley et al., 1992; Thomas and Rose, 1993; Carr, 1997). However, as with the previously considered factors the impact this may have is inconclusive, with Cohen (1980) reporting no correlations between any prior experiences or expectations of pain and the actual pain reported, and Walmsley et al. (1992) and Carr (1997) reporting positive although varying degrees of correlation.

Culture

Cultural differences complete the range of variables that are commonly suggested as key determinants of individual variance in the experience of pain. Early work by Zola (1966: 628) suggests that, when reporting conditions to a physician, a 'socially conditioned selective process may be operating'. Zola (1966: 616) remarks, specifically on differences between Irish and Italian patients and their reports of pain for the same condition, that 'it is striking that the pattern of response can vary with the ethnic background of the patient'.

Davitz et al. (1976, 1977a, 1977b) looked extensively into the impact of culture, not only on the individual's perception and reporting of pain but also on the impact cultural background may have on healthcare professionals' perceptions of others' pain. The bulk of their work confirmed that some form of cultural stereotyping seemed to exist between the different ethnic groups studied, and this is confirmed by the subsequent work of Streltzer and Wade (1981), Greenwald (1991) and Edwards et al. (2001), with Streltzer and Wade (1981: 402) concluding that, in the 'milieu (environment) of under-treatment of pain, some cultural styles are more susceptible to under-treatment than others'.

Consequently, although various factors are recognized as influencing the individual pain experience, the extent and interrelationship (if any) by which they do so remain unclear. This leaves sufferers and carers with many difficulties in the interpretation and appraisal of the pain experience.

The recognition of pain

The importance of recognizing and managing pain is well documented. There is a clear ethical obligation for all healthcare professionals to act in their patients' best interests, which must include the necessity of alleviating both pain and suffering wherever possible (Lisson, 1987; Greipp, 1992; Copp, 1993). Consequently the need to recognize, assess and manage pain, whether from the pain sufferers' or healthcare workers' perspective, is undisputed. However, it is equally indisputable that the ability of health-care professionals to do so is far below that required.

Within the community the incidence of pain is very difficult to gauge as reporting is haphazard and difficult to coordinate; however, figures for the UK suggest that the uncertainty in factual reporting of pain is itself a clear indicator of the lack of recognition that currently exists in all facets of pain appraisal and management.

Documentation

This picture of lack of recognition of pain is compounded by an equal fail-ure to document reported pain in either nursing or medical records. This was first reported by Camp (1987), who observed that less than 50% of pain assessments from a sample of 84 patients taken from medical, surgical and oncology settings were documented. Not only that, but of those that *were* actually documented less than 50% were congruent with a pain assessment of that patient carried out not more than 10 minutes later by the researcher. Camp was forced to conclude that 'nurses have not found pain sufficiently important to merit complete assessment and documentation' (Camp, 1987: 594). (See also Chapter 5.)

Albrecht et al. (1992) reported that nurses believed they documented pain much more frequently than they did in reality, with few perceiving the importance of documenting pain at all. Clarke et al. (1996) audited nursing documentation and found that 76% of charts had no documentation of pain assessment. Carr (1997) reported that, even after an extensive pilot of a pain assessment tool and care plan, 44% of patient evaluations did not include any references to pain. MacLellan (1997) reported that 77% of patients had no documentation of pain on record in either medical or nursing notes beyond 'analgesia given', and Meurier (1998), in an audit of pain assessment for patients with myocardial infarctions, found that all areas of pain documentation were inadequate, with assessment at a very superficial level where it takes place at all.

Discrepancies between nurse and patient assessments

This lack of recognition of pain is also illustrated in the discrepancies that occur between pain sufferer and healthcare professional where actual documentation of pain does take place. Iafrati (1986), in a small study of the correlation between nurses' and their patients' assessment of pain, found that 31% correctly assessed their patients' pain, 34.5% underestimated it, and 34.5% overestimated it. Choiniere et al. (1990) in a larger study of 42 patients and nurses reported correct assessments at 30%, underestimation at 43% and overestimation at 27%. Zalon (1993), in a study of 119 registered nurses and patients, found that only 34.5% of pain assessments were accurate, whereas nurses underestimated the amount of pain their patients reported in 45.4% of cases and overestimated in only 20.2%.

Healthcare professionals themselves reveal considerable awareness of the problems with recognition of pain. Fox (1982) found that 65% of nurses surveyed felt inadequate in their management of pain. Von Roerin et al. (1993), in a survey of 899 medical staff based in the eastern states of the USA, found that 86% believed that pain was undermedicated. Lloyd (1994) found that 70% of nurses believed that they underestimated patient's pain. This picture is also reflected in the extensive need for education to achieve appropriate pain recognition and management.

The under-recognition of pain

When discussing the factors that contribute to the under-recognition of pain at their simplest level they can be divided into two main areas: factors that prevent or exacerbate the communication of pain by the sufferer, and factors that prevent or exacerbate healthcare professionals' difficulties in recognizing pain.

The sufferer

Only limited numbers of studies specifically consider under-recognition of pain by sufferers, although some studies do report that, in some instances, considerable differences exist between sufferers' expectations of pain and relief and those of healthcare professionals.

Carr (1990) reports a continuing dichotomy between sufferers' and healthcare professionals' expectations about pain, including the belief from sufferers that nurses would recognize when they were in pain and give them analgesia accordingly although, in contradiction, nurses believed that sufferers should report pain to them so that they could then treat it. Linked to this, evidence in Carr's study suggests that, even if on questioning sufferers stated they would report pain to a nurse, in practice few of them appeared to do so.

It becomes apparent that sufferers may not always be helpful in assisting carers in the recognition of pain. Ferrell et al. (1991) found that 17% of nurses, as a reason for less than adequate pain recognition, as well as 35% of nurses reporting problems with the patient and their family as a further barrier, cited lack of cooperation from sufferers. Von Roenin et al. (1993) reported similar findings, with 62% of doctors surveyed stating that patient reluctance to report pain was a major barrier to recognition, compounded by reluctance among sufferers to take analgesics when prescribed. Juhl et al. (1993) reported that only 64% of 191 postoperative patients would inform staff if they were in pain, and Clarke et al. (1996) indicated that patient barriers to adequate pain recognition were a more important factor in the under-treatment of pain than nurses' knowledge or education about pain.

Mackintosh (1994b) and Carr (1997) both attempt to identify what the barriers may be that prevent sufferers from always cooperating or reporting pain, and conclude that many sufferers use minimizing techniques towards their own pain. These include concepts such as the belief that others are worse off than themselves, fear of further medical interventions including injections and opioid drugs, and minimal expectations of pain relief. This is also evidenced by a number of studies that report high incidence of unacceptable levels of pain, coupled with high levels of patient satisfaction with the pain management they have received (Cohen et al., 1980; Weis et al., 1983; Mackintosh and Bowles, 1997).

Whatever specific causal factors are evidenced it is apparent that sufferers themselves have some part to play in the under-recognition and subsequent poor appraisal of pain, and that their participation and cooperation is essential in order to ensure that sufferers received optimum care (Watt-Watson and Stevens, 1998).

Healthcare professionals

Numerous factors have been cited as responsible for under-recognition of pain by healthcare professionals; these include:

- inappropriate knowledge about pain;
- lack of appropriate education on pain for healthcare professionals;

- difficulties of communication;
- professional carer characteristics.

Inappropriate knowledge about pain

Virtually every study that has identified difficulties in the recognition, assessment and management of pain has also highlighted areas of knowledge deficit held by healthcare professionals, and indicates this as partly responsible for the poor quality pain care received by sufferers. Early studies, including the works of Cohen (1980) and Fox (1982), found that nurses held exaggerated fears about opioid addiction, made irrational choice of analgesic drugs and had inadequate knowledge of how analgesics worked.

Hamilton and Edgar (1992), with a sample of 318 qualified nurses, continued to find that fear of addiction remained a major constraint to appropriate use of opioid analgesia. Nurses remained unclear about the properties of opioids and were uncertain of the differences between acute and chronic pain. This lack of knowledge about analgesics is also a recurrent theme in many subsequent studies, including Mackintosh (1994a), McCaffery and Ferrell (1995), Carr (1997), Howell et al. (2000) and Mackintosh and Bowles (2000). Clarke et al. (1996) also found that nurses lacked knowledge of non-pharmacological pain interventions, the use of adjunctive medications, and the anatomy and physiology of pain.

Lack of appropriate education on pain for healthcare professionals

Education in appropriate methods of recognizing, assessing and managing pain has been regarded as a key factor in improving quality of care received by sufferers, and this would seem to be an obvious solution to many of the difficulties identified above. Weis et al. (1983) clearly identified education as a possible solution to the clinical problems identified in his study, as do Van Roenin et al. (1993), McCaffery and Ferrell (1995) and Mackintosh and Bowles (2000).

This is further supported by the work of Wilson et al. (1992), Dalton et al. (1996), McCaffery and Ferrell (1997) and Howell et al. (2000), who all demonstrate improvements in attitudes and knowledge towards sufferers of pain and pain management by healthcare professionals, following specific pain education programmes, whilst Clarke et al. (1996) showed a significant correlation between the higher level of nurse's education and the most accurate knowledge about pain recognition.

However, knowledge does not necessarily result in positive changes in practice. Lack of change in clinical behaviour towards sufferers of pain has been reported in studies where high levels of accurate knowledge concerning pain and its management were present (Dalton et al., 1996, 1998; Howell et al., 2000), with Langeveld et al. (1997) reporting that, although levels of knowledge about pain among the 174 nurses surveyed were good, this was not reflected in clinical interventions used, and that level of nurses' education had no impact on this finding.

Difficulties of communication

Communication is a fundamental part of the ability to recognize and appraise pain. However, the effectiveness and efficacy of healthcare professionals' communication skills have been constantly challenged and appear to be an ongoing source of stress, friction and anxiety for both healthcare professionals themselves and those they care for (Jarrett and Payne 2000; Lloyd et al., 2000).

These communication difficulties all have a significant impact on the recognition of pain. If healthcare professionals cannot communicate effectively with those they care for, then their ability to recognize pain, assess it and manage it must be severely constrained.

Professional carer characteristics

The final key area that has been linked with the consistent pattern of under-recognition of pain concerns the professional characteristics of healthcare professionals themselves (Harrison, 1991). These include factors such as the clinical setting in which professional carers work (Camp, 1987; Pitts and Healey, 1989), the length of time working in the healthcare profession (Choiniere et al., 1990; Lander, 1990; Hamers et al., 1994), and the medical diagnosis or the presence of pathology in the pain sufferer (Halferns et al., 1990; Short et al., 1990; Hamers et al., 1994). However, these factors are mainly inconclusive; other studies indicate only minimal differences in appraisal of pain as a consequence of professional experience (Halferns et al., 1990; Field, 1996a).

It becomes apparent that a vast range of factors may be responsible for the consistent and continuing difficulties in the appraisal of pain that result in the under-recognition, which has been extensively reported above. Individually these factors all have varied and uncertain levels of impact on the pain experience, but taken together they produce a considerable cumulative effect, all resulting in a consistent trend towards the under-recognition of pain, the lack of pain appraisal and subsequent poor management of pain.

The appraisal of pain

In order to overcome many of the above factors, which severely limit the recognition and subsequent appraisal of pain, it is good practice to adopt an objective and methodical approach to the appraisal and assessment of pain (Von Roenin et al., 1993; Field, 1996b; Mackintosh and Bowles, 1997). As Dunn (2000) argues, the formal assessment of an individual's pain conveys three essential meanings to the person in pain.

1. That the individual's complaint of pain is believed.
2. That the pain is being taken seriously.
3. That carers want to know what the pain is like for the person experiencing it.

It is, however, essential to emphasize that assessment cannot and should not be used to either prove or disprove whether reported pain is actually present as no objective determining measure of pain currently exists (McCaffery and Pasero, 1999). Formal assessment is also essential as an aid to successful management as 'without accurate pain assessment, pain will not be relieved successfully and the efficacy of different pain treatments cannot be measured' (Thompson, 1989: 149).

Pain should be assessed at a number of stages: initially after first onset (where possible) so that a full baseline assessment can take place, against which subsequent treatments can be measured; at suitable intervals following any interventions or treatments; and following any reported change in the sufferer's pain (Dunn, 2000).

Pain assessment can take a number of different forms, all dependent on the needs of the individual experiencing the pain, as well as the needs of the healthcare professionals attempting to appraise and manage it. However, key factors in assessment are essential in all areas of pain appraisal and management, and should be applied in practice wherever possible even in the swiftest and most urgent pain assessment.

The assessment of chronic pain also has some additional features, which are as a direct consequence of its nature:

- pain is a disease;
- it has an ill-defined onset;
- the pathology is often unidentifiable;
- there is absent or adapted pathology;
- there are peripheral central changes in somatosensory cortex;
- there is no known biological function;
- pain does not respond to treatment;
- it is associated with depression;
- it does not work well with the medical model;
- it involves the family, social network and lifestyle;
- the pain exists by itself and not merely as a symptom;
- its timespan is vague and unpredictable;
- appraisal does not depend on an established pathology;

- pain has no purpose;
- appraisal must go beyond efficacy of treatment;
- appraisal must include psychological state;
- appraisal must go beyond the medical model;
- appraisal should cover all relevant aspects of the sufferer's life.

Consequently the appraisal of chronic pain may have more levels of complexity than pain in its simple acute form. However, the key factors in assessment remain unchanged.

Key factors in assessment

Six key factors are commonly identified as the basic essentials of all pain assessment (McCaffery and Pasero, 1999; Dunn, 2000). These are:

1. Location. Where the pain is, or if multiple pain sites are present where they all are. (Individual pain sites should be assessed separately as they may all be different.)
2. Description. What each pain is like – hot, burning, stabbing. This may be a useful indicator of the cause of the pain, and it may also be useful to identify words the sufferer uses to label their own pain.
3. Duration. How long the pain has been present, as well as factors that trigger it off, and any variations in the pain so far.
4. Intensity. How much the pain hurts. This may be quantified in a number of ways either by simply recording the sufferer's own words or by using a formal pain assessment tool.
5. Influencing factors. Those factors that either aggravate or help relieve the pain – for example, position, temperature or activity.
6. Previous treatment. What may have worked for the same or similar pain in the past?

These key factors can be used in a number of different ways but most commonly as the basis for direct questioning of the individual pain sufferer. They also form part of the basis of a number of different pain-assessment tools and can be encompassed in a formal manner when used together with a recognized assessment tool.

Pain-assessment tools

A wide range of pain-assessment tools is currently available. As yet there is no one pain-assessment tool that meets the needs of every individual experiencing pain, or every clinical area, and it may be necessary to use a combination of tools for the individual pain sufferer as well as be familiar with a range of tools for each clinical area. As Dunn (2000) argues the key element is to use a tool that is readily understandable by the person with pain, rather than hold to a specific format.

The majority of pain-assessment tools all use the sufferer's self-report as the determining factor. These can be used only when the sufferer is capable of reporting the pain him- or herself, and this self-report should be considered the *gold standard* as the measure of the sufferer's pain (McCaffery and Pasero, 1999).

The commonest and most frequently used brief self-report pain-assessment tools are: descriptive scales, numerical scales and visual analogue scales (VAS). These scales are used almost exclusively to measure the intensity of the individual's pain. These scales are generally considered as easy and quick to use, understandable by most pain sufferers and carers, and flexible enough to be used in a variety of clinical situations with some consistency with use over time (Fordham and Dunn, 1994; Scott, 1994; Hawthorn and Redmond, 1998; McCaffery and Pasero, 1999; Main and Spanswick, 2000).

Examples of commonly used pain-assessment tools

Descriptive scales usually consist of a range of words describing pain on a continuum ranging from 'no pain' to 'unbearable pain'. These may be verbal scales used in an oral manner, or they may be available on paper for sufferers to indicate where their pain actually is.

The words used to describe the pain may be predetermined – mild, moderate and severe pain – or the sufferer's own words can be used.

Numerical scales work on a similar principle asking sufferers to describe the intensity of their pain in numbers rather than words, with a common scale of 0 = no pain and 10 = unbearable pain. These scales may be used orally, but are most commonly used in a written paper form, with either a horizontal or a vertical line, normally 10-cm long. Scales may be left blank with only defining numbers at each end, or may be marked at equal intervals along their length. Different numbers may also be used, for example 0 to 5 or 0 to 100.

Visual analogue scales, also known as graphic rating scales, follow the same principle asking the sufferer to indicate the intensity of their pain on a line, which is marked at either end only, usually with 'no pain' at one end and 'unbearable pain' at the other. The line may be horizontal or vertical. Sufferers are then asked to place a mark on the line indicating roughly where they believe their pain currently is.

Faces rating scales work on the same principle, but rather than using words or numbers instead represent the intensity of the pain experienced in a pictorial manner normally using faces, with faces ranging across the scale on a continuum from smiling to grimacing and crying. Of these the

Wang–Baker scale is the commonest, most frequently used for children or for adults who may have difficulty conceptualizing their pain as a word or number (Wang and Baker, 1988).

It is important to stress that brief assessment tools are reliant on self-report, are mainly used to assess one dimension of the pain experience and its intensity, and offer only a very superficial and limited interpretation of the sufferer's pain. For these to be used effectively they should form only one part of a fuller holistic individual assessment, which addresses all of the six key factors identified above.

In order to overcome the limitations of these brief pain-assessment tools a range of more complex and frequently multidimensional tools is also available. Again these are heavily reliant on self-report as the key determining factor but cover a wider range of factors affecting the pain experience. These are less flexible in their application as they may take considerable time to complete and are most frequently used in the assessment of chronic pain.

The McGill Pain Questionnaire is perhaps the best known complex tool; first developed in 1971, it uses a complex range of scoring categories to identify the individual's pain score. It has subsequently been developed in a brief form; this assessment tool remains largely within the remit of the chronic pain clinic assessment. It has been largely replaced by a number of other complex tools, which are more clinically focused and have a simpler structure for both the user and the healthcare worker.

The Initial Pain Assessment Tool is advocated by McCaffery and Pasero (1999) as providing a detailed initial assessment that incorporates all six key factors of appraisal, as well as providing a documented record of this appraisal, with the addition of a drawing of the human body, which can be used to mark the location of the pain as well as any movement. This has been successfully used in a variety of clinical areas where the nature of the pain allows an in-depth initial assessment to take place.

A similar complex tool is the Pain Audit Collection System (PACS), which incorporates measures of pain intensity with measures of functional/behavioural abilities to create the Brief Pain Inventory (BPI); this may also be used to audit the efficacy of treatment interventions. The simplicity and brevity of this tool have resulted in its increasing popularity, especially for the assessment of chronic pain (Pain Society, 1999).

Either of these tools may also be used in conjunction with a variety of other assessment tools (including the brief assessment tools discussed above), all considering different aspects of the pain experience; these may include measures of functional ability such as the Oswestry Disability Index, as well as measures of mood or psychological state including the Hospital Anxiety and Depression (HAD) index. It is important to note that the more complex the form of pain assessment the more time-consuming it is for both sufferer and healthcare worker, and this can lead to frustration and confusion, as well as resulting in more complex difficulties of interpretation by both the sufferer and the healthcare professional.

Pain assessment, where self-report is unavailable for whatever reason, is always complex and unreliable and should be avoided wherever possible. Studies of pain sufferers with degrees of cognitive impairment all suggest that simple pain tools such as numerical and descriptive rating scales should be initially attempted and may be useful in a variety of conditions, which may not be predictable (Fanurik et al., 1998; Delac, 2002). Where these measures are utterly inapplicable it may be possible to use behavioural tools as a potential indicator of disturbances in behaviours that may be triggered by unrecognized pain but these can be used only in long-term or chronic pain situations (Feldt et al., 1998a, 1998b, 2000). Consequently where assessment of pain is virtually impossible, pain should be treated in the same manner as is considered best practice for any individual with a similar complaint (Manfredi et al., 2003).

Problems with pain assessment tools

It is possible to argue that the inadequacy of these tools and the cumbersome nature of their use may be a major preventive to their widespread acceptance and use (Harrison, 1991; Field, 1996a; Meurier, 1998; Bell, 2002), and, even where extensive resources and education have been involved in the introduction of pain assessment tools into clinical practice, findings have been disappointing (Carr, 1997). There is also a body of evidence that suggests that many healthcare professionals do not use them as they are simply disliked as inaccurate, unnecessary, time-consuming encumbrances, or that healthcare professionals prefer to use their own personal subjective assessments (Nash et al., 1993; Hamers et al., 1994; Meurier, 1998; McCaffery et al., 2000).

These difficulties with pain assessment, compounded by the highly subjective and variable nature of the pain they are attempting to assess, ensure that formal documented assessment of pain remains to a large degree haphazard and of uncertain purpose.

Conclusion

The appraisal of pain is a complex, multifaceted process determined by the highly individual and subjective nature of pain itself. Yet accurate holistic appraisal of pain is essential for the pain sufferer in order to act not only as an aid for diagnosis and treatment but to ensure that the sufferer's pain is treated in a manner that conveys both belief and respect for their individual pain experience.

Pain appraisal involves many aspects: the individual variations in the experience for the sufferer as well as individual variations both personal and professional. The art and skill of appraisal involve drawing all these elements together to create an holistic individual assessment that is as accurate and objective as possible, to form a firm basis for successful treatment and management, providing the highest levels of care possible. Measuring pain is a key to treating it. Pain measurement is not just for clinical trials, nor even for audit. It should be something done regularly, like taking a temperature or measuring blood pressure (Moore et al., 2003).

References

Albrecht MN, Cook JE, Riley MJ et al. (1992) Factors influencing staff nurse's decisions for non-documentation of patient response to analgesia administration. Journal of Clinical Nursing 1: 243–51.

Bell F (2002) A review of the literature on the attitudes of nurses to acute pain management. Journal of Orthopaedic Nursing 4: 64–70.

Briggs E (2003) The nursing management of pain in older people. Nursing Standard 17(18): 47–53.

Burns JW, Hodman NBA, McLintock TTC et al. (1989) The influence of patient characteristics on the requirements for post-operative analgesia. Anaesthesia 44: 2–6.

Bush F, Hawkins SW, Harrington WG et al. (1993) Analysis of gender effects on pain perception and symptoms present in temporomandibular pain. Pain 53: 73–80.

Camp LD (1987) Comparison of medical, surgical and oncology patient's descriptions of pain and nurses documentation of pain assessments. Journal of Advanced Nursing 12: 593–8.

Carr ECJ (1990) Postoperative pain: patients' expectations and experiences. Journal of Advanced Nursing 15: 89–100.

Carr ECJ (1997) Evaluating the use of a pain assessment tool and care plan: a pilot study. Journal of Advanced Nursing 26: 1073–9.

Chambers WG, Price GG (1967) Influence of nurse upon effects of analgesics administered. Nursing Research 16: 228–33.

Choiniere M, Melzack R, Girard N et al. (1990) Comparisons between patient's and nurse's assessment of pain and medication efficacy in severe burn injuries. Pain 40: 143–52.

Clarke EB, French B, Bildeau ML et al. (1996) Pain management knowledge, attitudes and clinical practice: the impact of nurse characteristics and education. Journal of Pain and Symptom Management 11: 18–31.

Cohen FL (1980) Post surgical pain relief: patient's status and nurses medication choices. Pain 9: 265–74.

Copp LA (1974) The spectrum of suffering. American Journal of Nursing 74: 491–5.

Copp LA (ed.) (1985) Pain, ethics and the negotiation of values. In Perspectives in Pain: Recent Advances in Nursing. Edinburgh: Churchill Livingstone.

Copp LA (1993) (ed.) An ethical responsibility for pain management. Journal of Advanced Nursing 18: 1–3.

Crow S, Olivet LW, Burry Stock J et al. (1996) Assessment of pain coping styles: development of an inventory. Journal of Advanced Nursing 24: 890–8.

Dalton JA, Blau W, Carlson J et al. (1996) Changing the relationship among nurses' knowledge, self reported behavior and documentary behavior in pain management: does education make a difference? Journal of Pain and Symptom Management 12: 308–19.

Dalton JA, Carlson J, Mann JD et al. (1998) An examination of nursing attitudes and pain management practices. Cancer Practice: a Multidisciplinary Journal of Cancer Care 6: 115–24.

Davitz LJ, Sameshima Y, Davitz J (1976) Suffering as viewed in six different cultures. American Journal of Nursing 76: 1296–7.

Davitz LL, Davitz JR, Higuchi Y (1977a) Cross-cultural inferences of physical pain and psychological distress. 1. Nursing Times April: 521–3.

Davtiz LL, Davitz JR, Higuchi Y (1977b) Cross-cultural inferences of physical pain and psychological distress. 2. Nursing Times April: 556–8.

Degenaar JJ (1979) Some philosophical consideration on pain. Pain 7: 286–304.

Delac K (2002) Pain assessment with cognitive impairment is possible. Topics in Emergency Medicine 24: 52–4.

Donovan M, Dillan P, McGuire L (1987) Incidence and characteristics of pain in a sample of medical surgical inpatients. Pain 30: 69–78.

Dunn V (2000)The holistic assessment of the patient in pain. Professional Nurse 15: 791–3.

Edwards LL, Fillingim RB, Keefe F (2001) Race, ethnicity and pain. Pain 94: 133–7.

Fanurik D, Koh J, Harrison RD et al. (1998) Pain assessment in children with cognitive impairment: an exploration of self report skills. Clinical Nursing Research 7: 103–24.

Feine JS, Bushnell MC, Mien D et al. (1991) Sex differences in the perceptions of noxious heat stimuli. Pain 44: 255–62.

Feldt KS (2000) Improving assessment and treatment of pain in cognitively impaired nursing home residents. Annals of Long Term Care 8(9): 36–42.

Feldt KS, Ryden MB, Miles S (1998a) Treatment of pain in cognitively impaired compared with cognitively intact older patients with hip fractures. Journal of the American Geriatric Society 46: 1079–85.

Feldt KS, Warne MA, Ryden MB (1998b) Examining pain in aggressive cognitively impaired older adults. Journal of Gerontological Nursing 24: 14–22.

Ferrell BR, Eberts MT, McCaffery M et al. (1991) Clinical decision-making and pain. Cancer Nursing 14: 289–97.

Field L (1996a) Factors influencing nurses analgesia decisions. British Journal of Nursing 5: 838–44.

Field L (1996b) Are nurses still underestimating patients' pain postoperatively? British Journal of Nursing 5: 778–84.

Fordham M, Dunn V (1994) Alongside the Person in Pain. London: Baillière Tindall.

Fox LS (1982) Pain management in the terminally ill cancer patient: an investigation of nurses' attitudes, knowledge and clinical practice. Military Medicine 147: 455–60.

Griepp ME (1992) Under medication of pain: an ethical model. Advances in Nursing Science 15(1): 44–53.

Greenwald HP (1991) Interethnic differences in pain perception. Pain 44: 157–63.

Haley WE, Turner JA, Romano JM (1989) Depression in chronic pain, patient's relation to pain, anxiety and sex differences. Pain 23: 337–43.

Halferns R, Evers G, Abu-Saad H (1990) Determinants of pain assessment by nurses. International Journal of Nursing Studies 27(1): 43–9.

Hamers JPH, Abu-Saad HH, Halferns RJG et al. (1994) Factors influencing nurse's pain assessment and interventions in children. Journal of Advanced Nursing 20: 853–60.

Hamers JPH, Abu–Saad HH, Vanden Hout MA et al. (1996) The influence of children's vocal expressions, age, medical diagnosis and information obtained from patients as nurses pain assessments and decisions regarding interventions. Pain 55: 53–61.

Hamilton J, Edgar L (1992) A survey examining nurses knowledge of pain control. Journal of Pain and Symptom Management 7: 18–26.

Harrison A (1991) Assessing patient pain: identifying reasons for error. Journal of Advanced Nursing 16: 1018–25.

Hawthorn J, Redmond K (1998) Pain: Causes and management. Oxford: Blackwell Science.

Hayward J (1975) Information – A Prescription Against Pain. London: Royal College of Nursing.

Howell D, Bulter L, Vincent L et al. (2000) Influencing nurse's knowledge attitudes and practice in cancer pain management. Cancer Nursing 23: 55–63.

Iafrati NS (1986) Pain on the burn unit: Patient versus nurse perceptions. Journal of Burn Care and Rehabilitation 7: 413–16.

International Association for the Study of Pain, Subcommittee on Taxonomy (1979) Pain terms: a list with definitions and notes on usage. Pain 6: 249–52.

Jarrett NJ, Payne SA (2000) Creating and maintaining 'optimisms' in cancer care. International Journal of Nursing Studies 31(1): 81–90.

Juhl IU, Christensen BV, Bilow HH et al. (1993) Post-operative pain relief, from the patients' and nurses' point of view. Acta Anaesthesiologica Scandinavia 37: 404–9.

Lander J (1990) Clinical judgements in pain management. Pain 42: 15–22.

Langeveld N, Molenkamp C, Merks J (1997) Pain in children with cancer: knowledge and attitudes of Dutch paediatric nurses. Journal of Cancer Nursing 1: 171–6.

Lay TD, Puntillo KA, Miaskowski CA et al. (1996) Analgesics prescribed and administered to intensive care cardiac surgery patients. Does patient age make a difference? Progress in Cardiovascular Nursing 11(4): 17–24.

Lisson EJ (1987) Ethical issues related to pain control. Nursing Clinics of North America 22: 649–59.

Lloyd G (1994) Nurse's attitudes towards management of pain. Nursing Times 90(43): 40–3.

Lloyd G, Skarratts D, Robinson N, Reid C (2000) Communications skills training for emergency department senior house officers – a qualitative study. Journal of Accident and Emergency Medicine 17: 246–50.

McCaffery M (1983) Nursing the Patient in Pain. London: Harper & Row.

McCaffery M, Ferrell BR (1995) Nurses knowledge about cancer pain: a survey of five countries. Journal of Pain and Symptom Management 10: 356–69.

McCaffery M, Pasero C (1999) Pain: Clinical Manual. St Louis, MO: Mosby.

McCaffery M, Ferrell BR, Pasero C (2000) Nurses personal opinions about patient's pain and their effect on recorded assessments and titration of opioid doses. Pain Management Nursing 1(3): 79–87.

Mackintosh C (1994a) Non-reporting of cardiac pain. Nursing Times 30(90): 13, 36–9.

Mackintosh C (1994b) Do nurses provide adequate post-operative pain relief? British Journal of Nursing 3: 342–7.

Mackintosh C, Bowles S (1997) Evaluation of a nurse led acute pain service. Can Clinical Nurse Specialists make a difference? Journal of Advanced Nursing 24: 30–7.

Mackintosh C, Bowles S (2000) The effect of an acute pain service on nurse's knowledge and beliefs about post-operative pain. Journal of Clinical Nursing 9: 119–26.

MacLellan K (1997) A chart audit reviewing the prescription and administration of analgesia and the documentation of pain after surgery. Journal of Advanced Nursing 26: 345–50.

Main CJ, Spanswick CC (2000) Pain Management: An Interdisciplinary Approach. Edinburgh: Churchill Livingstone.

Manfredi PL, Breuer B, Meier DE et al. (2003) Pain assessment in elderly patients with severe dementia. Journal of Pain and Symptom Management 25(1): 48–52.

Mather L, Mackie J (1983) The incidence of post-operative pain in children. Pain 15: 271–82.

Melzack R, Abbott PV, Zackon W et al. (1987) Pain on a surgical ward: a survey of the duration and intensity of pain and the effectiveness of medication. Pain 29: 67–72.

Meurier CE (1998) The quality of assessment of patients with chest pain: the development of a questionnaire to audit the nursing assessment record of patients with chest pain. Journal of Advanced Nursing 27: 140–6

Moore A, Edwards J, Barden J et al. (2003) Bandolier's Little Book of Pain. Oxford: Oxford University Press.

Nash R, Edwards H, Nebauer M (1993) Effect of attitudes, subjective norms and perceived control on nurse's intention to assess patient's pain. Journal of Advanced Nursing 18: 941–7.

Pain Society (1999) PACS. Clinical Information Special Interest Group. London: The Pain Society.

Pitts M, Healey S (1989) Factors influencing the inferences of pain made by three health professions. Physiotherapy Practice 5: 65–8.

Royal College of Surgeons and Royal College of Anaesthetists (1990) Commission on the Provision of Surgical Services: Report of the Working Party on Pain after Surgery. London: RCS/RCA.

Sanders SH, Brena SF, Spier CJ et al. (1992) Chronic low back pain patients around the world, cross cultural similarities and differences. Clinical Journal of Pain 8: 317–23.

Scott IE (1994) Effectiveness of documented assessment of post-operative pain. British Journal of Nursing 3: 494–501.

Short LM, Burnett ML, Egbert AM et al. (1990) Medicating the post-operative elderly: how do nurses make their decisions? Journal of Gerontological Nursing 16(7): 12–17.

Streltzer J, Wade TC (1981) The influence of cultural groups on the under treatment of post-operative pain. Psychosomatic Medicine 43(5): 397–403.

Strong J (1999) Chronic Pain: The Occupational Therapists' Perspective. Edinburgh: Churchill Livingstone.

Taezner P, Melzack R, Jeans ME (1986) Influence of psychological factors on postoperative pain, mood and analgesia requirements. Pain 24: 331–42.

Thomas VJ, Rose FD (1993) Patient controlled analgesia: a new method for old. Journal of Advanced Nursing 18: 1719–26.

Thomas V, Health M, Rose D et al. (1995) Psychological characteristics and the effectiveness of Patient Controlled Analgesia. British Journal of Anaesthesia 74: 271–6.

Thompson C (1989) The nursing assessment of the patient with cardiac pain in a coronary care unit. Intensive Care Nursing 5(4): 147–54.

Umlauf RL (1992) Psychological interventions for chronic pain following spinal cord injury. Clinical Journal of Pain 8: 111–18.

Von Roennin JM, Cleeland CS, Gonin R et al. (1993) Physician attitudes and practice in cancer pain management: a survey from the Eastern Cooperative Oncology Group. Annals of Internal Medicine 119: 121–6.

Walmsley PN, Brockopp DY, Brockopp GW (1992) The role of prior pain experience and expectations on post-operative pain. Journal of Pain and Symptom Management 7: 34–7.

Wang D, Baker L (1988) Pain in children: a comparison of assessment scales. Paediatric Nurse 14: 9–17.

Watt-Watson J, Stevens B (1998) Managing pain after coronary artery bypass. Journal of Cardiovascular Nursing 13(3): 39–51.

Weis OF, Sriwatanakul K, Alloza JL (1983) Attitudes of patients, housestaff and nurses towards post-operative analgesic care. Anesthesia and Analgesia 62: 70–4.

Weisenberg M, Caspi Z (1989) Cultural and educational influences on pain of childbirth. Journal of Pain and Symptom Management 4: 13–19.

Wilson JF, Brockopp GW, Kryst S et al. (1992) Medical students' attitudes towards pain before and after a brief course on pain. Pain 50: 251–6.

Wittink H, Michel TH (1997) Chronic Pain Management for Physiotherapists. Boston, MA: Butterworth-Heinemann.

Zalon ML (1993) Nurse's assessment of post-operative patients' pain. Pain 54: 329–34.

Zola IK (1966) Culture and symptoms – an analysis of patients presenting complaints. American Sociological Review 31: 615–30.

CHAPTER FIVE

Barriers to effective pain management

ALISON GRAY

Aims

- To explore beliefs and attitudes held by healthcare professionals that could present a barrier to effective pain management.
- To explore patients' and families'/carers' beliefs and expectations regarding pain management that could present a barrier to effective pain management.
- To explore how the healthcare system as a whole can affect pain management.

Objectives

- To understand why pain can be undertreated due to the beliefs and attitudes shared by healthcare professionals and patients.
- To challenge current practices in order to improve the patient's condition and reduce the pain they experience.
- To understand the nurse's role in facilitating change through challenging beliefs, assumptions and misconceptions.

Introduction

The under-treatment of pain has been repeatedly highlighted in the nursing press, yet with the wide range of medications and interventions available the question remains: 'What prevents pain from being managed effectively and why?'

This chapter seeks to explore how the beliefs and attitudes of health professionals and the patients and families they come into contact with affect the management of pain within the hospital environment. It will question why 'Barriers are treated as merely clinical failures, free of any significant

113

moral implications' (Rich, 2000) rather than as an ethical and moral obligation that needs addressing in terms of why some people suffer needlessly. Procedures are also suggested that may be developed and put in place to minimize or prevent pain. These issues will be examined and debated by taking an in-depth look at relevant research and literature, and highlighting examples from the author's own clinical experience.

Definition

It is important to recognize what is meant by the term 'a barrier to effective treatment' and, more specifically, the term 'barrier'. A barrier might be defined in two ways: first as something that prevents access (in the physical sense) and, second, as an obstacle to communication. Subdivisions of the definition include a drawback, a hindrance or a stumbling block. All are relevant here. The obstacle might be caused through misconception or misinformation (communication), or by the structure of the health service and its affiliates as such (physical).

Background

The administration of analgesia is a task that the majority of nurses will take part in every day of their working lives. As the healthcare professional in closest contact with the patient (Raiman, 1986; Caunt, 1992), the nurse is in an ideal position to use his or her skill and professional knowledge to relieve suffering and distress. Despite ongoing research and investigations into techniques employed in this field, findings continue to report that pain is poorly controlled in the hospital environment. One can also assume this is true within the community setting.

Davies (1996), Allcock (1996), Lloyd (1994) and Mann and Redwood (2000) highlight the under-treatment of pain as something that still happens regularly within the hospital setting. If a goal of nursing is to assist the patient to have the highest level of independence and functionality regardless of the underlying condition (Zimmerman et al., 1996), then nurses should more regularly examine and reassess their role and clinical practice in order to achieve an acceptable standard of nursing care that will fulfil this goal.

A study of the literature on pain management in the more general nursing press shows that very little of it touches on the ethical considerations of allowing patients to experience pain but some studies nevertheless conclude that if patients suffer needlessly this should raise ethical concerns for the medical staff involved (Montes-Sandoval, 1999). Closs (1990) states that 'unnecessary suffering should not be permitted simply on humanitarian grounds'. In order to find in-depth articles covering this subject more specialist journals need to be investigated – see, for example, Rich (2000).

It could be argued that, in failing to treat patients with pain adequately, the nurse is not fulfilling her duty as outlined in the Code of Professional Conduct (UKCC, cited in Edwards, 1996). For example, clause two of the code states that the nurse must: '[E]nsure that no act or omission on [his/her] part . . . is detrimental to the . . . safety of patients and clients' (UKCC, 1992, cited in Edwards, 1996).

Edwards (1996) states that this clause is in keeping with the ethical principle of non-maleficence, which is the obligation not to cause harm to others. The experience of pain can cause physiological harm and psychological damage to the patient (Caunt, 1992; Carson and Mitchell, 1998). Inadequate treatment suggests the code is being contravened and questions the degree of responsibility and intervention shown by the nurse to the patient.

Hawthorn and Redmond (1998: 87) list common reasons for unrelieved pain as follows.

Fault with healthcare professionals

- Poor knowledge about the nature of pain and its management.
- Poor pain assessment:
  - Inadequate collection of data
  - Poor recognition of the multidimensional nature of pain
  - Poor timing of assessment
  - Poor interpretation of data
  - Underutilization of pain assessment tools
  - Poor documentation.
- Poor utilization of pain-management skills.
- Myths and misconceptions about opioids:
  - Fear of addiction and respiratory depression
  - Fear of tolerance
  - Misconceptions about the placebo response
  - Ageism.

Fault with patients and family members

- Reluctance to report pain:
  - Desire to be a 'good' patient
  - Fear of addiction with opioids
  - Fatalistic attitudes about pain management
  - Belief that pain builds character
  - View pain as having moral value

- Non-compliance with treatment.
  - Lack of understanding
  - Desire to maintain some control of the situation
  - Belief that analgesic agents should only be taken when absolutely necessary
  - Belief that strong pain medication should be saved until the pain gets really bad.

Fault with the healthcare system

- Barriers to opioid availability:
  - Bureaucratic regulations about prescribing opioids
  - Unwillingness of pharmacies to stock opioids.
- Breakdown in continuity of care:
  - Poor system of organizing nursing work
  - Poor coordination of care between different healthcare settings
  - Low priority given to pain management
  - Lack of accountability for pain management.

The healthcare professional

Whether we, as nurses, like it or not, our beliefs and values affect every action we make, and will have an impact on those within our care, whether positive or negative. These perceptions can influence and be passed on to those we mentor and teach. In light of this it is therefore vital that these feelings and beliefs are explored, understood and possibly reconsidered in order for them not to adversely affect those within our care. As Loveman and Gale (2000) state, 'a key role in the assessment of patient pain and its remediation is the perception of the patient's pain by the nurse'.

Many theories have been put forward to explain the assumptions that some nurses make when treating the patient in pain. One of the most detailed is that researched by Davis (1988), where he lists 16 assumptions that nurses must grade on a scale as to whether they strongly agree with the assumption or strongly disagree with it, or judge it on the levels in between. The format used in this study has been replicated in some form or other by other researchers (Scott, 1992; Hunt, 1995; Mackrodt, 2001) and results continue to indicate that misconceptions and false beliefs are in evidence in the clinical arena.

Hawthorn and Redmond (1998: 97) summarize myths and misconceptions held by healthcare professionals about pain and its management as follows:

- all pains have an identifiable physical cause;
- people with the same tissue damage should experience similar levels of pain;
- patients who are sleeping are not in pain;
- patients who are in pain will let the nurse know about it;
- some pains (such as cancer pain) are inevitable and intractable;
- opioids should be reserved until the pain is really bad;
- non-pharmacological interventions are only effective for mild pain;
- patients taking opioids on a prolonged basis become addicted;
- the use of opioids for pain is associated with clinically significant respiratory depression;
- patients who come from areas where drug abuse is a common problem are more likely to become addicted;
- pain relief following placebo injection indicates that patients are lying about their pain;
- elderly patients experience less pain than younger people;
- infants do not experience pain.

Nurses feel that they have to justify their analgesic choices

Wakefield (1995) conducted interviews with five nurses and discovered that they were more likely to administer analgesia if they could establish a cause for pain as if needing to justify their professional choices. The discovery that nurses felt that they had to verify what the patient said rather than taking their statements at face value (Thorn, 1997) is a matter of some concern. Perhaps this is due to the subjective nature of pain, and a perception of how much pain an individual should experience in any given situation. There is also the problem of facing questions from other nurses or colleagues who may have felt that the choice of treatment was too strong or too weak.

Case study 1

Nurses are discussing a patient who continually asks for additional analgesia for backache of an unknown cause. Once the co-dydramol has been given and the pain still persists, the senior nurse questions if the pain really warrants something stronger, as this is just backache, and the patient is not exhibiting many signs of obvious distress.

Thought: Does a patient need to be constantly changing position in bed, or cold and clammy and in obvious distress, before analgesia is administered? Is medication the only intervention that this patient may need? What signs do you expect to see in order to intervene with medication? Is the patient's verbal report sufficient?

Perhaps the need to justify analgesia administration stems from the suggestion made by some nurses that patients may publicly display activity associated with discomfort to obtain additional medication (Wakefield, 1995), or to draw compassion and assistance from others (Montes-Sandoval, 1999), and therefore the nurse needs to be absolutely convinced of need in order to administer treatment. The implication is that patients may develop behaviour patterns to manipulate a desired response. The vitally important aspect of nurses' role in pain management is to believe patients, rather than assuming that they know how they are feeling, how effective medication is for them, or having preconceived and judgemental ideas about the rationale behind their behaviour. Madjar (1999) points out the need for carers not to doubt the reality of a person's pain but to acknowledge its existence. The often-quoted definition of pain from McCaffrey and Beepe (1994) supports this nursing action: 'Pain is whatever the experiencing person says it is and exists whenever he says it does.' Nurses need to be aware of the dangers of dismissing the patients' emotions, believing them to be secondary in status to their own erroneous truth (Wakefield, 1995).

Nurses fear opioid addiction

Many articles in nursing literature highlight the 'exaggerated beliefs about the addictive properties of opiates' (Closs, 1990). Lloyd (1994) also suggests that nurses have a fear of opioid addiction, and Willson (2000) suggests that fears about opioids hinder their administration. The term 'opiophobic' has been coined to describe those healthcare professionals who are unwilling to administer opioids (Hofland, 1992). Morgan (1985) interprets this as the irrational and undocumented fear that appropriate use of opioid drugs causes addiction. Despite the wealth of information that clearly indicates that there is a less than 1% chance of addiction when administering opioids for pain management (McCaffrey and Beebe, 1994), in articles that have been published for some years these fears still abound.

Fears about becoming dependent upon medication, causing respiratory depression and having difficulty in ever ceasing to require certain drugs, are very apparent throughout conversations with both healthcare professionals and lay people. These range from people not wanting to take too many tablets, to concern about the long-term effects of the stronger analgesic choices. However, opioids, when used for the right reasons, are certainly beneficial and will enhance a person's life and ability to live it. In order for something to be life threatening it does not have to threaten one's existence – it can adversely affect the ability to live life and to do the things needed to be done or, in this case, to feel free from discomfort and or distress.

Case study 2

Mr Kent has been receiving diamorphine for pain since admission to hospital. The frequency with which he asks for it is increasing. Nursing staff are now showing reluctance to administer the medication as they fear that he is developing tolerance and becoming dependent on the medication as he shows little sign of being in pain for most of the time.

Thought: The idea that Mr Kent feels better now that his pain is relieved is not considered. It is not seen as an achievement that his pain is now more controlled and that with some fine adjustments to dosages he may be able to have a pain-free existence. Ulterior motives are suspected. In addition, being judgemental about what should constitute an acceptable level of distress before analgesia is administered means that we are waiting for pain to be suffered before giving treatment, rather than attempting to relieve these painful episodes in the first place.

Pain needs to have an identifiable cause

It has been suggested that nurses are more likely to administer analgesia if the cause of the pain is known (Wakefield, 1995). However, much research has illustrated that, even in the surgical setting, pain is not always given optimal treatment, despite an obvious cause. Patients report that pain is not relieved (Cohen, 1980; Weis et al., 1983). Yet under these more controlled circumstances the pain should be more easily defined and a rationale behind the administration of analgesics be given and documented. It is important to note that pre-existing conditions causing chronic pain will continue to cause discomfort and require treatment appropriate to that need, as could something as uncomplicated as a headache caused by the stress of undertaking a surgical procedure. Some clinical areas use flow charts to enable more accurate assessment and administration of medication, thus providing a clearer set of guidelines for nurses and doctors to follow. However, assessing pain will have value only when increasing the effectiveness of interventions made. In addition, some authors see charting as a problem. Carson and Mitchell (1998) suggest that they may actually prevent nurses from really understanding the patient's experience of pain, and that 'a sincere commitment on the nurse's part to listen, comfort and act when required may be a more helpful approach'.

The steady evolution of modern technology has provided us with many answers to important questions that were previously impossible to answer. Even so, there are still many that remain unanswered and, in spite of our new-found knowledge, we must accept that much more needs to be done.

For a long time to come we shall be faced with pain caused by conditions that are not obvious or even identified during the course of an illness, but we must remember that these feelings are real to patients and have an adverse effect on their quality of life.

Nurses question the patient's right to be pain free

In one study, 400 questionnaires were sent to nursing staff and 269 replied. Of these, 28% of day staff and 44% of night staff expected their patients to experience pain, whereas 70% accepted that they underestimated pain (Lloyd, 1994). In comparison, Bowman (1994), after interviewing 16 patients and 13 nursing staff, discovered that the level of pain was incorrectly assessed 89% of the time, with 78% of nurses underestimating pain level.

Previous studies that have used the nursing assumptions' questionnaire of Davis (1988) have reported mixed feelings about pain management. Scott (1992) also discovered this in her study, finding that 41% of qualified staff were unsure about or even opposed to the right of a patient to a pain-free existence. Hunt (1995) found that 24 out of 35 nurses considered that they were better qualified to assess a patient's pain than the patients themselves.

Obviously, goals set for monitoring pain management need to be both measurable and achievable. It would be unrealistic to assume that all pains can be relieved immediately. For instance, the first goal may be to alleviate pain overnight, and reduce it during the day, or to reduce pain on movement but to be pain free at rest. Patients will need to be aware that not all pains can be relieved completely, but they should take encouragement from knowing that, whatever is prescribed, the goal will always be to work towards the improvement of their quality of life. It will need to be recognized that it may take several attempts for the pain to be managed effectively but also that there is no question of anyone resigning themselves to the view that pain is to be expected, and therefore unavoidable.

A duty of care is placed in the hands of registered nurses (McKane, 2000) but this is of little use if people continue to suffer needlessly. The inability to manage pain can even be interpreted as negligence. In the USA, a health-care provider was held liable for failing to treat pain in a patient who was terminally ill. The family was awarded $US15 million in damages (Davies, 1996). Unfortunately, this was too late to improve the comfort of the patient.

Case study 3

'Well, he's bound to experience some discomfort, he's just had major surgery. Just tell him to keep pressing on the patient-controlled analgesia (PCA) when he needs to – that should help.'

Thought: Is this a sufficient response? What response might you make to a patient who is experiencing pain following surgery and who suffers already with chronic pain? If you were the patient, what would you want to be told? Is it acceptable to expect pain following surgery? Is morphine the only pain relief that should be offered after surgery, or might a combination of analgesia help?

Why patients do not request improved standards

In light of the above, the question arises as to why patients do not ask for, or demand, improved standards of care. Perhaps they are conditioned by many of the same assumptions and are therefore contributing to the barriers, which also exist. However, there may be more subtle differences.

Expecting to experience pain

Just as nurses may expect patients to experience pain, perhaps patients also expect this and are not aware that their pain may be being under-treated (Rich, 2000). As Mann and Redwood (2000) explain, if patients are admitted to hospital expecting to experience pain, and they consequently do so, they can still say that they are satisfied with the level of care they received. As Closs (1990) elaborates, some patients will believe that pain should be endured, for example, as something they expect from having had surgery.

Does this indicate a lack of understanding and awareness on the part of patients or does it reflect their cultural and social beliefs? Hofland (1992) argues that if patients have been 'socialized in a culture that stressed stoicism, they may rarely complain of pain, as it would be considered a sign of weakness'.

Moreover, many people do not spend extended periods of time in hospital, or have training and knowledge equivalent to those looking after them. They have no way of knowing if the pain that they are feeling is to be expected or not. They rely entirely on the wisdom of the professional staff who care for them.

The hospital environment

A hospital provides an environment with which the nurse is familiar; however, this will probably not be the case for the patient. People enter hospital with their own perceptions and expectations, based on prior experiences and earlier memories. They may have once been patients themselves, or they might have visited a relative in hospital, or they might have been affected by someone else's experiences in hospital. Whatever they may have been, all of these can influence how the person reacts, responds and consequently behaves in hospital.

It has been suggested that life as a patient on a hospital ward can be threatening. People may find themselves in an unfamiliar environment, surrounded by people who are not yet known to them, and might be expected to adhere to the demands and expectations of the hospital routine while not necessarily feeling at all well. Anxiety can arise as people lose their identity through wearing hospital nightclothes and by being identified by a wrist label (Raiman, 1986) culminating in, for some, the adoption of the 'passive role' because they do not want to appear troublesome or for fear of being labelled a 'bad patient' (Hofland, 1992). Closs (1990) and Hofland (1992) both suggest that patients often do not inform staff of the existence or severity of the pain although they may, in fact, be willing to discuss it, because they perceive that the nurses are too busy and they do not want to take up their time. Admirable as this might appear, more often than not it leads to increasing demands on the patients' resources for dealing with the pain and a consequent decrease in their physical and psychological state.

Nurse–patient relationship

Patients and their families require additional support and time if a meaningful decrease in the amount of pain experienced is to result from the treatment administered. The therapeutic relationship should focus on establishing an environment in which trust and honesty will prevail and where patients and nurses are on an equal footing. For example, although when at home a patient may have responsibility for taking analgesia as required, in the hospital situation medications are locked away and taken only with the agreement of the nurse. In Heyes' (1999) research participants stated that they felt the need to 'convince' the assessing person that they had pain in order to be given analgesia, illustrating how an unequal balance of power in a relationship can occur and can be maintained. In addition, discussions about a patient's fears can elicit valuable information. Something such as a fear of needles, or a previously unpleasant experience with a certain drug, can cause a patient to deny the existence of pain. If the fear is known then a nurse can use an alternative route of administration or a different drug. This can be achieved only through honest and consistent dialogue between the healthcare professional and the patient.

In order for a consistent, forward-thinking approach to occur, the relationship between the nurse and the patient needs to be established and built upon so that both parties can move towards the same goal. If the patient's needs are ignored or not recognized it is to the detriment of the relationship that has been built.

Equally, education for nurses, patients and their families can lead to increased cooperation, and should result in improved standards of care. For example, patients in one study felt that, had they received prompt attention and interventions from the staff looking after them, then their pain could have been eased, rather than becoming a problem for them (Mann and Redwood, 2000). However, this will happen only if patients feel that they can relate concerns immediately and know that they will be acted upon. If this is not done, patients whose pain is not relieved will begin to feel increasingly anxious and may lose confidence in their families and the staff looking after them (Raiman, 1986).

It has been suggested that providing sufficient pharmacological intervention within a reasonable amount of time is one method that a nurse can use to gain the patient's trust (Cornock, 1996). As Hofland (1992) highlights, if patients have cause to believe that the nursing staff are not accepting what they say to be true, appearing too hurried or 'abrupt', they may resort to under-reporting how they are feeling. On the other hand, if patients understand the treatment regimen, they are less likely to feel frustrated and more likely to feel that they are in control.

Healthcare system

Inevitably, the system within which we work will have an effect on the standard and quality of care offered and, even if education focuses on relieving myths and preconceptions surrounding pain management, relevant procedures also need to be put in place to address the issue of poor pain management in the hospital and community setting. The system must support raising the priority level of this type of nursing intervention. Willson (2000) found that 'time, organisation of care, influence of shift worked and impact of the multi-disciplinary team' all affected the administration of analgesia to the patients in her study, with time causing concern in all areas. She argued that education alone will not be enough to increase standards and quality of care and that all of these areas need to be addressed in their entirety in order for change to be effective.

Obviously there are numerous factors that affect the healthcare system as a whole, and it would be impossible to discuss them all. They range from funding, staff shortages, government priorities and resources, to pressure on length of stay in hospital arising from patients and lack of hospital beds. The items discussed below are those that nurses could face on a daily basis and that we need to strive to overcome.

The hierarchical nature of the nursing environment means that junior nurses may develop behaviours based on what their senior counterparts do and teach. Their senses are constantly bombarded by the thoughts and feelings of others. If a senior nurse questions, or even just makes a comment, about whether or not certain medications should be administered, the junior and student nurses will become part of an environment where they are aware of false assumptions and misconceptions, may even believe them to be true, and consequently may incorporate them into their everyday practice.

If this is combined with inadequate nurse education in this area, as has been highlighted in research (86% of nurses in one study did not feel that their basic training prepared them to nurse the patient in pain – Fothergill-Bourbonnais and Wilson-Barnett, 1992), then it would be correct to assume that when confronted with misconceptions the nurse may not have sufficient theoretical knowledge to know if they are wrong. If supposition rather than theory is incorporated into practice at this stage then misconceptions threaten to dominate the working environment.

Ritualistic practice

Books on nursing rituals have highlighted the 'task orientation' of the drug round (Walsh and Ford, 1995). An ethnographic study carried out by Willson (2000) documents results of semi-structured interviews and participant observation concerning the routine administration of medication. She describes how, in an orthopaedic trauma unit, pain assessment was carried out at the same time as the drug round.

Case study 4

Nurse Smith is doing the lunchtime drug round. As she does so she reaches Mr Saunders who has received 'as required' analgesia for the last three drug rounds. She asks 'Are you in any pain?'. 'Yes nurse – the leg still hurts', for which he receives the prescribed dose of co-proxamol. Nurse Smith moves on to the next patient.

Thought: The example illustrates how, in completing one task (administering a drug), the nurse has established that Mr Saunders is in pain but has not done anything to evaluate if previously administered analgesia has been effective. The need to relieve pain has become secondary in importance to the general task-orientation pattern of the ward. What action could the nurse have taken to improve Mr Saunders' pain management?

In nursing education, the nursing process is highlighted as one that begins with assessment, leading to the nurse being able to plan, implement and evaluate care (Royle and Walsh, 1992). This should be an ongoing process as individual needs may change on a day-by-day basis. Care should be evaluated and then re-evaluated. The nursing process should be implemented repeatedly throughout the patient's stay.

The need for thorough pain assessment to be incorporated into practice has been raised in an earlier paper by Walker and Campbell (1988, cited in Baillie, 1993) when they state 'Pain assessment and control should be a priority within nursing'. If adequate time is not put into carrying out all parts of the nursing process interventions made may well be less effective.

Pain-assessment tools

One method by which pain can be addressed thoroughly and effectively is through the use of assessment tools. Despite being widely available, they appear to be inconsistently applied in practice (Willson, 1992) or not available at all. Managing change in any environment is challenging, as people can resist, due to fear of change, or because they feel that an already exhausting workload is about to increase yet again.

However, such tools will be of value only if misconceptions on the part of the nurse do not lead to inaccurate assessments (Fothergill-Bourbonnais and Wilson-Barnett, 1992). Research studies have shown that 'administration of analgesia often bore no relation to recorded pain assessment' (Lloyd, 1994).

Case study 5

We often hear the phrases 'not more paperwork – that's all I do these days' and 'I just don't have time!' It is sometimes perceived to be easier to resist change, as it will inevitably require reorganization of the workload and shifting the focus of behaviours. It can also, however, provide the stimulus to increase satisfaction in the quality of nursing care and the lives of those with whom we come into contact.

Controlled drug administration

In addition to the concerns surrounding the administration of opioids 'the time and manpower it takes to administer controlled opioids may also influence the decision as the procedure takes the time of at least one nurse'

(Willson, 2000). In some hospitals, due to the need for two nurses to administer controlled drugs, it is less easy to administer medication, and this frequently means there is a delay in meeting patients' needs. This dilemma was recognized by Mann and Redwood (2000), noting that procedural requirements were causing a significant delay in the administration of opioids. In order to improve the standard of patient care, the 'two-nurse administration' requirement was removed. Although appearing to be a good idea in theory this may be counterproductive as it places greater responsibility on the nursing staff because decisions are made in isolation, as opposed to being taken after discussion with and agreement from a fellow professional.

Conclusion

It would appear that the most difficult aspect of the management of pain is its subjective nature. Feelings are so individual and personal that it is only through establishing dialogue between patients and staff that any inroads can be made into eliminating and managing a person's pain. The basis of all these nursing interventions always will be, and should be, through effective communication.

We can identify numerous obstacles that need to be overcome before pain can be properly and appropriately managed in all healthcare environments. These originate from patients and staff and from procedures that are currently in place. It will only be through openness and a willingness to change, and through being prepared to accept and operate different strategies and educational approaches, that standards will improve and barriers will be broken down for the patients within our care.

References

Allcock N (1996) Factors affecting the assessment of postoperative pain: a literature review. Journal of Advanced Nursing 24: 1144–51.

Baillie L (1993) A review of pain assessment tools. Nursing Standard 7(23): 25–9.

Bowman JM (1994) Perception of surgical pain by nurses and patients. Clinical Nursing Research 3(1): 69–76.

Carson MG, Mitchell GJ (1998) The experience of living with persistent pain. Journal of Advanced Nursing 28: 1242–8.

Caunt H (1992) Reducing the psychological impact of postoperative pain. British Journal of Nursing 1: 13–19.

Closs SJ (1990) An exploratory analysis of nurses' provision of postoperative analgesic drugs. Journal of Advanced Nursing 15: 42–9.

Cohen FL (1980) Post-surgical pain relief: patients' status and nurses'medication choices. Pain 9: 265–74.

Cornock M (1996) Psychological approaches to cardiac pain. Nursing Standard 11(12): 34–8.

Davies K (1996) Findings of a national survey of acute pain services. Nursing Times 92(17): 31–3.

Davis PS (1988) Changing nursing practice for more effective control of postoperative pain through staff initiated educational programme. Nurse Education Today 8: 325–31.

Edwards SD (1996) Nursing Ethics – A Principle-based Approach. London: Macmillan.

Fothergill-Bourbonnais F, Wilson-Barnett J (1992) A comparative study of intensive therapy unit and hospice nurses' knowledge on pain management. Journal of Advanced Nursing 14: 362–72.

Hawthorn J, Redmond K (1998) Pain Causes and Management. Oxford: Blackwell Science, pp. 87, 97.

Heyes ML (1999) Teaching pain management: how to make it work. Journal for Nurses in Staff Development 15(1): 27–36.

Hofland SL (1992) Elder beliefs: blocks to pain management. Journal of Gerontological Nursing June: 19–24.

Hunt K (1995) Perceptions of a patient's pain: a study assessing nurses' attitudes. Nursing Standard 10(4): 32–5.

Lloyd G (1994) Nurses' attitudes towards management of pain. Nursing Times 90(43): 40–3.

Loveman E, Gale A (2000) Factors influencing nurses' inferences about patient pain. British Journal of Nursing 9: 334–7.

McCaffery M, Beebe A (1994) Pain – Clinical Manual for Nursing Practice. London: Mosby.

McKane M (2000) Research, ethics and the data protection legislation. Nursing Standard 14(20): 36–41.

MacKrodt K (2001) Nurses' knowledge within the context of pain management. Journal of Orthopaedic Nursing 5(1): 15–21.

Madjar I (1999) On inflicting and relieving pain. In Nursing and the Experience of Illness. London: Routledge.

Mann E, Redwood S (2000) Improving pain management: breaking down the invisible barrier. British Journal of Nursing 9: 2067–72.

Montes-Sandoval L (1999) An analysis of the concept of pain. Journal of Advanced Nursing 29: 935–41.

Morgan JP (1985) American opiophobia: customary underutilization of opioid analgesics. Advances in Alcoholism and Substance Abuse 5: 163–73.

Raiman J (1986) Towards understanding pain, and planning for relief. Nursing 3(11): 411–23.

Rich BA (2000) An ethical analysis of the barriers to effective pain management. Cambridge Quarterly of Healthcare Ethics 9: 54–70.

Royle JA, Walsh M (1992) Watson's Medical Surgical Nursing and Related Physiology. London: Baillière Tindall.

Scott I (1992) Nurses' attitudes to pain control and the use of pain assessment scales. British Journal of Nursing 2(1): 11–16.

Thorn M (1997) A survey of nurses' attitudes towards the assessment and control of postoperative pain. Journal of Orthopaedic Nursing 1: 30–8.

Wakefield AB (1995) Pain: an account of nurses' talk. Journal of Advanced Nursing 21: 905–10.

Walsh M, Ford P (1995) Nursing Rituals: Research and Rational Actions. Oxford: Butterworth-Heinemann.

Weis OF, Sriwatanakul K, Alloza JL (1983) Attitudes of patients, housestaff and nurses towards postoperative analgesic care. Anesthesia and Analgesia 62: 70–4.

Willson H (1992) Painful facts. Nursing Times 88(35): 32–3.

Willson H (2000) Factors affecting the administration of analgesia to patients following repair of a fractured hip. Journal of Advanced Nursing 31: 1145–54.

Zimmerman L, Turner-Story K, Gaston-Johansson F, Rowles JR (1996) Psychological variables in cancer pain. Cancer Nursing 19(1): 44–53.

CHAPTER SIX

Invasive techniques

Carol Banks

Aim

To introduce the reader to the use of invasive techniques for the management of chronic pain within the context of a multidisciplinary pain management service.

Objectives

By the end of the chapter the reader will:

- be able to appreciate and understand the rationale, timing, efficacy, contraindications and potential complications of invasive pain-management techniques;
- be aware of the various invasive pain-management techniques available, their appropriateness, limitations and benefits.

Introduction

Until the 1960s, pain clinics, pain specialists and pain research barely existed and pain was generally thought of as a byproduct of disease. It is reasonable to think of acute pain in this way but, today, professionals working in the field of chronic pain consider chronic pain as a specific healthcare problem and even a disease in its own right. Unlike acute pain, chronic pain often serves no biological purpose and causes a great deal of disability and suffering, not just for those in pain but also for people close to them.

Before the 1960s it was generally believed that the sensory nervous system was like a set of wires that conducted impulses from the periphery to the brain, rather like a telephone exchange system. It would be logical, then, to think that if a specific nerve is causing pain the surgeon should cut or destroy the offending nerve and terminate the painful sensation. If a nerve is cut or destroyed the pain is abolished, until the nerve regenerates and the pain returns. This could be due to the fact that the pathology that was in the nerve has migrated centrally into the spinal cord, where cells become hyperexcitable (see Chapter 2). This type of surgery is now rarely performed and used only when pain is severe and the life expectancy of the person is less than 6 months, although there is the odd exception to this rule such as destruction of the small nerves supplying sensation to the facet joints of the spine.

Over the last half-century many invasive procedures have been developed and used for the treatment of chronic pain, spurred by the publication of Melzack and Wall's gate-control theory of pain (Melzack and Wall, 1965). The gate-control theory provides a conceptual framework within which pain perception is explored and explained. The effect of this theory on pain research has been profound and has led to a greater understanding of the complexity of chronic pain from both a physiological and a psychosocial point of view, while also evoking researchers to take up the challenge of exploring the mechanisms of chronic non-malignant pain. Specific aspects of the gate-control theory have been challenged and modified over the years; however, the basic concept that transmission of painful information can be modulated has been supported by both experimental and clinical experience.

Patients in pain and other health professionals often ask for a 'nerve block' to be performed to abolish the pain sensation completely. This highlights a general lack of understanding about pain mechanisms, management strategies and the belief that a cure for chronic pain is simply at the end of a needle or surgeon's knife. There are times when this could be the case but generally it is not and it can be very unhelpful for patients who will have had their expectations raised only to have them dashed again. This can then lead to increased emotional distress, frustration, anger, depression and an increase of observed pain behaviour.

Neurodestructive techniques are now considered inappropriate for chronic non-malignant pain sufferers. A more pragmatic view has evolved among pain specialists, which encompasses the complex nature of the chronic pain experience. Pain clinics are not called 'pain relief clinics' but 'pain-management clinics', the emphasis being on management and not relief. Pain-management clinics make every effort to relieve pain but put equal effort into reducing a person's disability, distress and suffering. This can be done only when a multidisciplinary, systematic, biopsychosocial approach is used. These days most pain-management clinics offer a wide range of treatment strategies, the primary aim of which is to maximize the patient's quality of life. These treatments can be summarized into three categories:

1. medication;
2. psychologically based treatment;
3. invasive techniques.

These three treatment approaches are not mutually exclusive. A combination of different methods may be necessary to provide satisfactory pain relief. This will differ for each type of pain and each person in chronic pain.

Several different therapeutic and diagnostic invasive procedures are commonly used in most pain clinics. Although no one injection or block is a panacea or a total cure for chronic pain, when used within the context of a holistic, patient-centred approach, benefits to the patient's quality of life can be achieved. Although invasive techniques in pain management alone are rarely curative they can facilitate active participation in rehabilitation. Therefore they do have a role to play in the treatment of chronic pain but only when the pain is localized. Before any invasive procedure is undertaken patients should always be fully informed regarding complications, side effects, and any limited duration of action of the treatment that is planned as well as their role in active rehabilitation.

This chapter will focus on the role of invasive techniques that are used both therapeutically and diagnostically to help the person suffering chronic pain,

Chronic pain treatment continuum

The diagnosis and pathology of chronic pain are very complex and a single pathophysiological explanation is not always available for some patients, which is why most chronic pain clinics have a range of invasive and non-invasive procedures that can be used both therapeutically and diagnostically to help sufferers. The chronic pain continuum is not linear. The continuum, depending on the chronic pain sufferer's needs, can be entered or exited at any point. Generally the least invasive treatment interventions are tried first. The continuum shows a range of pain management strategies that a chronic pain clinic can provide (Figure 6.1).

Neuroablation

Implantable intraspinal opioids

Chronic strong opioids

Cognitive behavioural therapy

Cognitive behavioural programme

Implantable spinal cord stimulation

Corrective surgery

Tricyclic antidepressants, membrane-stabilizing drugs

Moderate-strength opioids

Neural blockade

Physical therapy

TENS/Acupuncture

NSAIDs and/or over-the-counter drugs

Figure 6.1 Pain-management strategies. NSAIDs, non-steroidal anti-inflammatory drugs; TENS, transcutaneous electrical nerve stimulation.

Searching for a pain source

Most patients presenting at a chronic pain clinic will already have undergone a plethora of investigations and/or operations in the hope of finding the source or cause of the pain. When a medical model of cause and effect is applied to chronic pain many patients can be subjected to unnecessary operations or investigations in the search for the source or origin of the pain impulse. Pain is primarily a subjective experience and therefore no test exists to objectively measure pain perception. Pain cannot be seen on an X-ray or a scan. For example, in over 85% of patients with lumbar and cervical pain no specific spinal pathology can be identified as the cause of pain (Bardense, 1999). In areas of medicine other than pain management little thought is given to the plasticity of the central nervous system, inhibitory pain pathways or central sensitization processes. This is partly due to the complexity of chronic pain syndromes and the lack of understanding of these processes by many health professionals. That said, every effort should be made to identify pathology that can be eliminated where possible.

Continued chronic back and/or leg pain following one or more spinal surgeries is an interesting example of how complex the search for a pain source can be. One of the problems that clinicians face when dealing with this complex group of patients is that the cause or causes of continued pain are not easily defined.

Long (1991) lists the following as some of the physiological generators of pain perception in chronic back and leg pain after spinal surgery:

- abnormalities of muscle, fascia and ligaments;
- myositis, fasciitis and bursitis;
- instability of the spine;
- compression of nerves;
- lumbar disc degeneration;
- disc bulging, without nerve compression;
- arthritic facet joints;
- scar tissue (fibrosis);
- epidural adhesions;
- arachnoiditis.

Examples of the psychosocial issues that can contribute to continued pain perception in people with chronic pain are:

- depression;
- fear of pain, leading to low activity;
- emotional distress;
- anxiety/stress/anger/frustration/low self-esteem/low mood;
- loss of role in family and society;
- physical deconditioning;
- social security issues;
- compensation issue;
- behavioural gain.

It is clear that patients presenting at a chronic pain clinic require a thorough biopsychosocial assessment. Timing and preparation of any invasive procedures need to be considered carefully as failure or further treatment failure could cause the person unnecessary emotional distress.

Neural blockade and other invasive chronic pain-management techniques

Anaesthetists frequently perform nerve blocks to modulate nociception to allow for pain-free surgery. Specialist pain doctors (SPDs) have taken this approach one step further and now frequently perform nerve blocks to modulate the pain sensation of chronic pain states. Nerve blocks are procedures that involve the administration of local anaesthetic agents, steroids or neurodestructive agents centrally (through the central nervous system) to visceral plexus or to peripheral nerves (peripheral nervous system) and muscle (trigger point injection). Sympathetic nerve blocks are performed at the stellate ganglion, celiac plexus, lumbar and thoracic sympathetic chain, and the ganglion impar. Sympathetic blocks are useful in visceral, vascular and sympathetically maintained pain. Advanced neuromodulation techniques involve the modulation of pain sensation within the central nervous system by the use of either medication into the intrathecal space or the placement of electrodes near to the spinal cord. Advanced neuromodulation techniques such as spinal cord stimulation (SCS) and intrathecal drug delivery are long-term strategies that are often undertaken in more specialist pain-management centres.

Invasive pain-management interventions can be divided into two groups: those that are diagnostic and those that are therapeutic. Some diagnostic blocks can lead to a therapeutic block. For example, the injection of facet joints with local anaesthetic, if successful, can lead to a procedure to destroy the small nerves that innervate the facet joints. The primary aim of neural blockade is to interrupt the neural input at its source. The objectives are as follows:

- to ascertain the specific pathway involved in the maintenance of the pain;
- to aid the differential diagnosis of the source/cause of continued pain;
- to determine the patient's reaction to the elimination of pain, and to the procedure.

Table 6.1 shows the main difference between diagnostic blocks and therapeutic blocks/interventions.

Table 6.1 Diagnostic block versus therapeutic block/intervention

Diagnostic blocks/intervention	Therapeutic blocks/intervention
Ascertain specific nociceptive pathways	Control of severe acute postoperative pain and pain from self-limiting disease
Help determine mechanism of chronic pain syndrome	Breaking of 'vicious' cycle involved in some pain syndromes may provide prolonged relief
Aid differential diagnosis of the site and cause of pain	Provide temporary relief to permit other therapies, or used in combination with other therapies
Determine patient response to pain relief and procedure	Neuroaugmentation of chronic pain (SCS, intraspinal drug delivery)

SCS, spinal cord stimulation.

Diagnostic blocks

Diagnostic blockade is used as part of 'an integrated diagnostic process', which can be useful in supplying the pain physician with information regarding both the mechanism of pain and the possible source of the pain by identifying the neural pathway that could be mediating the pain impulse, helping to define the anatomical correlates of the clinical pain disorder (Boas, 2002).

Examples of diagnostic blocks include:

- Local anaesthetic agents on the facet joints of the spine. Back and neck pain is particularly complex and can involve many structures. Therefore the injection of the facet joints can help either to eliminate the facet joints as a cause of continued pain or to aid the diagnosis of facet joint pain.
- Local anaesthetic agents in specific peripheral nerves such as the lateral cutaneous nerve or the trigeminal nerve, which can help differentiate between trigeminal neuralgia and atypical facial pain or musculoskeletal pain.

Therapeutic blocks/interventions

There are many procedures that can be used diagnostically within both the peripheral nervous system and the sympathetic nervous system. However, there are fewer procedures available that are considered therapeutic in that they remove, destroy or modulate the source of the pain. Nevertheless, there are occasions when long-term pain relief is achieved after a series of local anaesthetic blocks, so there are times when a series of local anaesthetic blocks could be considered diagnostic and therapeutic. Even if only short-term pain relief is achieved, this can sometimes allow the patient to increase activity and movement and 'break the pain cycle'. Advance neuromodulation can also be considered therapeutic in that long-term pain relief is the primary therapeutic goal of the treatment.

Outcome

The outcome of both therapeutic and diagnostic blocks depends not only on the measure of pain relief achieved but also patients' reaction to any reduction in their pain. It may seem odd to some that an SPD may also be as interested in the patient's response to the pain relief that is achieved following a block as in the pain reduction achieved. When a person has had chronic pain for a long time it often leads to inactivity and deactivation. Therefore it is important to assess how patients respond to pain relief. Do they become more active and start to exercise the affected area more easily? Or do they stay the same and make no effort to reactivate themselves physically? In other words, does the patient's pain behaviour change or not as a result of short-term pain reduction? Table 6.2 summarizes invasive procedures and whether they are diagnostic or therapeutic, where they are used and for what indication.

Table 6.2 Summary of invasive procedures

Procedure	Therapeutic or diagnostic	Structure (part of nervous system)	Drug used	Indication
Trigger point injection	Diagnostic and therapeutic	Peripheral nervous system	LA ± corticosteroid	Localized muscular pain
Peripheral nerve block	Diagnostic and therapeutic	Peripheral nervous system	LA ± corticosteroid	Peripheral neuralgia Radiculopathy
Facet joint injection Facet joint denervation	Diagnostic and therapeutic	Peripheral nervous system	LA ± corticosteroid or heat	Spinal pain
Epidural injection	Diagnostic and therapeutic	Peripheral nervous system	LA or corticosteroid	Dermatomal leg pain
Stellate ganglion block	Therapeutic	Sympathetic nervous system	LA	Refractory angina CRPS 1 and 2
Paravertebral block	Therapeutic	Sympathetic nervous system	LA	Refractory angina CRPS 1 and 2
Lumbar sympathectomy	Diagnostic and therapeutic	Sympathetic nervous system	LA	PVD CRPS 1 and 2
Intravenous sympathectomy	Therapeutic	Sympathetic nervous system	Guanethidine LA	CRPS
Spinal cord stimulation	Therapeutic	Central nervous system	Electrical stimulation	FBSS, CRPS, Refractory angina
Intrathecal drug delivery	Therapeutic	Central nervous system	Opioids Clonidine LA	Chronic malignant and non-malignant pain

CRPS, complex regional pain syndrome; FBSS, failed back surgery syndrome; LA local anaesthetic; PVD, peripheral vascular disease

Contraindications for invasive pain-management interventions

There are few contraindications for invasive pain-management techniques, the main one being that the patient is already taking anticoagulation medication, although this can be stopped for a few days prior to the procedure to avoid any unnecessary bleeding. Other contraindications include:

- lack of patient consent;
- clotting abnormalities;
- presence of local or systemic infection;
- psychological distress.

Local anaesthetic agents

Local anaesthetics agents (LAs) are sodium channel-blocking agents, which block unmyelinated C- and B-fibres and small myelinated A-delta-fibres with little or no interruption of motor function, although there are occasions when a motor effect is sought as in relief of severe muscle spasm. The block produced is reversible and does not damage nerve tissue. The duration of the effect depends on the concentration and type of LA used. The pain-relieving effects of LA blocks often last much longer than the pharmaceutical effects of the LA agent used.

Most side effects and complications relating to invasive pain-management techniques are related to the use of LAs. Therefore invasive pain-management procedures should be performed only in a clinical area where resuscitation equipment is readily available, intravenous access is achieved, and an image intensifier is used to ensure precise location of the needle before injection of the LA agent.

Side effects and complications

The most serious potential consequence of the use of LA agents is a systemic toxic reaction due to accidental injection of LA either intravenously or intrathecally. Hence the need for the precautions mentioned above. The symptoms of systemic toxicity of LA agents range from mild to severe. Mild effects include palpitations, dry mouth, vertigo and confusion. Severe effects include convulsions, severe hypotension, bradycardia, respiratory depression and cardiac arrest. Systemic effects of LA agents must be treated promptly. Preventive measures include always drawing back the syringe before injection and use of X-rays to aid needle placement.

Corticosteroids

The mechanism of analgesia produced by corticosteroids involves both an anti-inflammatory effect and a direct effect on electrical activity in damaged nerves (Devor et al., 1985). The commonest use of corticosteroid injections for chronic pain management is in the reduction of inflammatory arthritic joints, the aim being to reduce severe pain and increase mobility.

Corticosteroids are licensed for intramuscular and intra-articular use and injection into soft tissue. Corticosteroids are not licensed for epidural use but have commonly been used for this purpose for many years. The patient must be informed of the unlicensed use of a drug as part of the consent process.

Side effects and complications

The use of corticosteroids for inflammatory arthritis is limited because damage to the cartilage can occur after more than three intra-articular injections. Generally systemic side effects are avoided by the use of depot-steroid solutions, which only have an effect locally and not systemically.

Trigger-point injection

Myofascial pain is the most common cause of pain in a pain clinic, being responsible for around 55% of chronic head and neck pain and 80% of back pain (Aronoff et al., 1983).

A myofascial trigger point is a hyperirritable area of skeletal muscle that is associated with a hypersensitive palpable nodule in a taut band of muscle (Simon et al., 1999). The trigger point is painful when compressed and can also give rise to referred pain. Trigger points can be found in:

* muscles;
* fasciae;
* tendons;
* ligaments and joint capsules;
* periosteum;
* scars.

Trigger points can be caused by a number of factors including:

* trauma;
* repeated sprain;
* persistent muscle contraction caused by stress;

- prolonged immobility;
- repetitive micro-trauma.

For many years the recognized treatment for trigger points has been the local injection of local anaesthetic agents with or without corticosteroids. The trigger point is first located by palpation and the needle is inserted into the area of pain. The injection is given when pain is provoked. Trigger-point injections are considered both diagnostic and therapeutic: a good but short-term relief of pain will confirm diagnosis. In a more acute situation the short-term relief of pain may allow for free movement of the area, which can lead to 'breaking of the pain cycle'.

Indications

The injection of trigger points is appropriate only when one or two trigger points are isolated. When multiple myofascial trigger points are present, as seen in fibromyalgia, it would not be helpful to attempt to inject all of the trigger points present. Patients with fibromyalgia require a more holistic treatment regimen based primarily on education.

Evidence

It seems that, in appropriately selected patients, myofascial trigger point injections can be helpful in decreasing pain and improving range of movement when used in conjunction with a rehabilitative approach (Borg-Stein, 1996), and have been shown to be one of the most effective treatment modalities for the deactivation of trigger points.

Peripheral nerve blockade

The peripheral nervous system consists of 31 pairs of spinal nerves, 12 pairs of cranial nerves and the autonomic part of the nervous system.

Peripheral nerves can be blocked as they exit the spinal cord as for epidural injection or nerve root injection, as well as in the smaller branches. The peripheral nervous system includes both sensory and motor nerve fibres.

The primary purpose of neural blockade in both acute and chronic pain is to interrupt the nociceptive impulse at its source. Peripheral nerve blockade is primarily a diagnostic procedure due to the short duration of action of local anaesthetic agents. A specific nerve can be blocked using a local anaesthetic agent to determine and confirm the diagnosis. The neural blockade of peripheral nerves is a very useful diagnostic tool, which has several practical uses within a pain-management clinic. These are:

- confirmation of diagnosis by identifying a specific neural pathway as the source of pain;
- confirmation of a precise target area before proceeding to a more invasive technique;
- repeated short-term relief which can sometimes lead to more long-term pain relief;
- allowing for observation of the patient's response to short-term pain relief.

Indications

Peripheral nerve blockade is indicated when peripheral nerve damage is suspected and the pain is described in an area of a specific peripheral nerve innervation.

Blocks to spinal nerve structures

Probably the commonest peripheral nerve blocks used for chronic pain are those acting on the spinal nerves for the relief of nerve root pain.

Epidural injection

The epidural administration of an LA agent and corticosteroid solution is a common treatment for acute and chronic nerve root pain. The primary reason for an epidural injection is to reduce local inflammation and/or reduce nerve root irritation, caused by inflammatory chemicals from a prolapsed or degenerative intervertebral disc, which spill on to the nerve roots causing irritation and pain in a limb. The procedure is usually performed with the patient awake or sedated, in a prone position and with the aid of radiographic guidance to ensure correct placement of the drug.

Indications

An epidural injection involves the placement of the drug/drugs in the epidural space at the spinal level of the reported spinal pain, or the dermatomal level of nerve root pain. The indications for an epidural injection are:

- constant radiating pain in a leg/arm, which corresponds to the spinal level at dermatomes;

- signs of nerve root irritation, such as positive straight leg-raising test (reproduction of leg pain by raising the leg);
- signs of nerve root compression such as motor or sensory reflex deficits;
- magnetic resonance imaging (MRI) evidence of a herniated intervertebral disc at a level that corresponds to the symptoms.

The evidence

A meta-analysis performed by Watts and Silagy (1995) on the efficacy of epidural corticosteroids for the treatment of sciatica concluded that epidurally administered corticosteroids were effective at 6 months and 12 months in the management of lumbosacral nerve root pain of variable duration. However, there is no evidence for the effectiveness of epidural injection for low back pain alone.

The fact that around 80% of herniated discs will resolve in time and without the necessity for surgery means that an epidural injection can be helpful as it can allow the patient to resume activity and aid the recovery process.

Facet joint injections

The spinal vertebrae articulate to form three joints, one being the joint between the vertebral bodies and the other two being the right and left facet joints, which are formed between the superior and inferior articular processes of the vertebral bodies. The facet joints help to resist the sheering movement on forward flexion of the spine and the corresponding force of spinal rotation. Facet joint pain is the commonest cause of chronic pain following whiplash injury.

Blockade of the facet joints can be considered both a diagnostic and a therapeutic procedure. Local anaesthetic, with or without corticosteroids, is injected using radiographic guidance control to the small nerves that innervate the facet joints. If the block is successful then radiofrequency denervation (destruction of nerve supply) can be performed in order to achieve a much longer outcome. With the acceptance of the treatment of cancer pain with a limited life expectancy this is the only pain-relieving procedure that is neurodestructive.

Indications

The diagnosis of facet pain is still poorly defined; relief of pain following injection with an LA is probable the best indication. Some features of facet joint pain include:

- paravertebral tenderness;
- increased pain on lateral bending and spinal rotation;
- increased pain on spinal extension rather than flexion;
- straight leg-raise test not provoking pain;
- deep, aching spinal pain.

The evidence

The reported results of cervical facet joint injections seem to be favourable to those for the lumbar spine. There is some evidence that facet joint injections can reduce chronic pain of facet joint origin. The injection of the joints can help confirm a diagnosis before proceeding to nerve denervation. Therefore, as a diagnostic test, facet joint injections have proved to be valid (Bogdok and Lord, 1998).

Sympathetic blockade

The sympathetic nervous system normally regulates the amount of blood flowing through tissues, organs and sweat glands. In an emergency the fibres of the sympathetic nervous system change their action when their cell bodies are informed of damage causing increased activity of the sensory nerve fibres, as well as regulating blood flow. These fibres also play a part in triggering the inflammatory response from tissue damage.

The lateral chain of the sympathetic ganglia extends from the upper cervical level to the sacrum. Sympathetic blockade is used in chronic pain conditions that are thought to be sympathetically maintained and can be performed at prevertebral and paravertebral sympathetic ganglia, for example stellate ganglia and lumbar sympathetic ganglia. The injection of LA on to the section of the sympathetic trunk that innervates the affected area of the body interrupts nerve conduction in the sympathetic nerves. Blockade to the sympathetic nervous system is a component of any regional block including blocks to the spinal nerves, due to spread on to the sympathetic chain.

In the past an intravenous technique was used to achieve a sympathetic blockade for the treatment of complex regional pain syndrome type 1 (CRPS 1). Use of an intravenous regional technique with an adrenergic antagonist and an LA agent did this. Evidence now shows that this technique is not efficacious and its use has become rather controversial. The least controversial use of sympathetic blockade is for peripheral vascular disease (PVD) when the patient has severe pain at rest and is not a candidate for vascular surgery. These patients can proceed to a permanent sympathectomy in order to achieve long-term pain reduction and improved circulation to the affected limb(s).

The involvement of the sympathetic nervous system in the generation and/or maintenance of chronic pain is still poorly understood. However, it is known that the sympathetic nervous system plays a role in the maintenance of peripheral nerve pain. It is also responsible for the afferent pain sensation from the abdominal and cardiovascular systems and pelvic viscera.

Stellate ganglion block

The stellate ganglion is a star-shaped collection of nerve cells on the sympathetic chain at the root of the neck. A stellate ganglion block can be performed for the following chronic pain conditions:

- refractory angina pectoris;
- CRPS 1 of the upper limbs;
- CRPS 2 of the upper limbs;
- herpes zoster.

Thoracic perivertebral block

The paravertebral space is an anatomical space, much like an epidural space. The contents of the space include the mixed (sensory and motor) somatic nerve. There are also sympathetic efferent fibres passing with the nerve, which proceed to the sympathetic ganglion. Some fibres pass through the ganglion and pass up and down the sympathetic chain; others synapse in the ganglion. A paravertebral injection will spread on to the sympathetic ganglion and will spread up and down a few levels as well. Thus a somatic paravertebral block will, in the thoracic region where the sympathetic chain is more posteriorly placed, produce a segmental sympathetic block.

Thoracic perivertebral block is indicated for the following pain types:

- CRPS 1;
- CRPS 2;
- refractory angina pectoris;
- visceral pain – for example, pancreatitis.

Lumbar sympathetic nerve block is indicated for:

- PVD;
- phantom limb pain;
- stump pain;
- neuropathy;

- CRPS 1 of the lower limbs;
- CRPS 2 of the lower limbs.

Evidence

Clinical evidence indicates that a subgroup of patients with neuropathic pain do respond to sympathetic blockade. There is a lack of good quality randomized controlled trials to confirm the efficacy of sympathetic blocks.

Advanced neuromodulation

Spinal cord stimulation and intrathecal drug administration

Advanced neuromodulation includes two main therapies, which are invasive and costly and involve the implantation of devices. These include SCS and intrathecal (IT) drug delivery. Advanced neuromodulation should be used only when more conservative and less costly therapies have failed to provide relief of chronic pain and suffering, and within experienced specialist chronic pain centres.

Spinal cord stimulation provides neuromodulation of neuropathic and ischaemic pain, but not nociceptive pain. When used for appropriate indications in the right individuals it can provide up to 50–60% long-term pain relief in up to 50–60% of patients trialled for efficacy (Turner, 1995). Neuroaugmentation techniques include treatments such as transcutaneous electrical nerve stimulation (TENS), peripheral nerve stimulation (PNS), deep brain stimulation (PDS) and SCS.

The term 'intraspinal/intrathecal' encompasses delivery of drugs via the epidural and the intrathecal routes. Intrathecal drug delivery with opioids such as morphine or fentanyl or non-opioids such as clonidine and bupivacaine can provide pain relief in nociceptive, neuropathic pain and mixed pain states in patients who have had a successful trial of intraspinal drug delivery. As with most other chronic pain treatment strategies the goal of the treatment is not analgesia alone, but analgesia that facilitates and leads to active rehabilitation of the individual. Therefore it must be said that invasive long-term therapies for chronic pain management such as SCS and intrathecal drug delivery can be successful only when the patient is a partner with the pain-management team and where psychosocial and behavioural factors are always taken into account.

There are five phases of advanced neuromodulation treatment:

1. patient selection and screening/physiological and psychological;
2. patient and family education;

3. trial of IT medication and trial of SCS;
4. preoperative and postoperative care;
5. maintenance, long-term follow-up for review, and refill and trouble-shooting.

Careful patient selection and management are significant determinants of a positive outcome with advanced neuromodulatory techniques. This section will explore the process of patient selection and describe the intervention, complications, indications and efficacy within the context of the five stages of treatment.

Contraindications for advanced neuromodulation

The contraindications for advanced neuromodulation are:

* lack of patient consent;
* clotting abnormalities;
* presence of local or systemic infection;
* psychological exclusion criteria met.

Spinal cord stimulation

Spinal cord stimulation is a reversible non-destructive treatment for some types of chronic pain. It involves an electrical device consisting of implanted electrodes, connected by a lead to an implanted receiver or pulse generator. The lead is inserted into the epidural space percutaneously or in an open operation. The first SCS system was implanted in 1967. Since then the technology, the technique and guidance regarding indications for SCS have improved.

Spinal cord stimulation has developed as a direct consequence of the gate-control theory of pain, which proposes that afferent sensory fibres in the dorsal columns all send branches into the spinal cord dorsal horn, where they enter the spinal cord. Each electrical pulse applied to the dorsal columns sends impulses towards the brain, and other impulses descend and enter the dorsal horn, so the gate is closed by the stimulation of large-diameter fibre impulses. It is assumed that these impulses entering the dorsal horn trigger an inhibition in the pain pathway (Melzack and Wall, 1995), thereby closing the theoretical gate and preventing or reducing the potential for pain perception. Patients feel the stimulation-induced paraesthesia (Chapter 2) as a pleasant tingling sensation in the area of their pain.

Spinal cord stimulation also seems to activate several different mechanisms to treat different types of pain. In ischaemic pain, animal experiments demonstrate that inhibition of afferent activity in the spinothalamic tracts, long-term suppression of sympathetic activity and antidromic effects on peripheral reflex circuits may take place to alleviate the pain of ischaemia (Linderoth and Foreman, 1999).

Most SPDs who perform SCS implantation for chronic pain perform the operation in two stages.

The first stage is the placement of the lead containing the electrodes into the epidural space using radiological control for guidance. This is usually performed under LA to enable the patient to provide feedback to the SPD about where the tingling is felt. The aim is to produce stimulation-induced paraesthesia in the area of pain. The lead containing the electrodes is then attached to an extension cable and tunnelled under the skin about 15 cm from the entry site. Patients then have the opportunity to trial SCS for 1–4 weeks, allowing them to use SCS while undertaking everyday activities in their own environment. The outcome of the trial is considered positive if patients report a significant reduction in pain and an improvement in their quality of life.

Patients proceed to the second stage and a pulse generator or receiver is implanted, usually into the subcutaneous tissue of the abdomen. They are able to control the system using a hand-held programmer or a transmitter attached to the implanted receiver.

Indications for SCS

It is important that an accurate diagnosis of the underlying pain aetiology and type is made before SCS is considered for a patient. There is general agreement that SCS is a treatment for severe neuropathic pain such as radiculopathy and peripheral nerve lesions, and ischaemic pain conditions such as PVD and, most recently, refractory angina.

It has been shown to be particularly helpful in the relief of neuropathic pain states. These include CRPS types 1 and 2, cauda equina damage, peripheral neuropathy and deafferentation pain such as phantom pain and stump pain (Simpson, 1994). By far the commonest use of SCS is for 'failed back syndrome' when the leg pain is greater than the back pain (North, 1994). Failed back syndrome is often a mixed pain condition; the leg pain is frequently radicular and the back pain can be nociceptive in nature. In parts of America SCS is now used before spinal reoperation (North, 1994).

More recently SCS has been used as part of a treatment continuum for the treatment of refractory angina pain with excellent results. See www.angina.org for details of nursing guidelines and other information on this topic. If a patient with chronic stable angina does not respond to pharmaceutical and surgical management and is no longer a candidate for further revisualization surgery, SCS guidelines can be applied. The treatment continuum for these patients starts with counselling and progressing through to SCS implant. It is important to add that SCS does not mask the pain of myocardial infarction and is considered a safe and effective treatment for this group (Mannheimer et al., 1996).

Intrathecal drug administration

There are occasions when a person's chronic pain is resistant to more conservative chronic pain treatments but the pain responds to opioid medication. However, the experience of debilitating and troublesome side effects prevents the use of a therapeutic dose of oral opioid medication. These patients can be considered for intrathecal drug delivery via an implanted pump.

Intrathecal drug delivery uses an implantable drug delivery system to administer very low doses of opioid or other analgesic into the intrathecal space, thereby saturating the opioid receptors. The dose required to achieve an analgesic effect is much lower than that needed for systemic administration. Continuous intrathecal opioid delivery provides a stable cerebrospinal concentration of opioid drug.

Intrathecal drug delivery is an invasive procedure that requires continued follow-up, for pump refills and evaluation of the treatment. It is not a treatment option that is considered lightly. The patient needs to be fully informed and included in the decision-making process. A trial of IT therapy is always conducted before the implantation of a pump – the trial can be epidural or intrathecal, continuous infusion or by intermittent bolus delivery. The outcome of the trial is judged by pain relief achieved and the patient's response to a reduction in pain.

The delivery of opioids directly into the intrathecal space avoids the unwanted systemic effects of oral or parental opioids, as the drug is targeted at the point of their action in the central nervous system. Therefore direct infusion of opioids or non-opioids offers the following advantages:

- potent analgesic response;
- stable therapeutic drug levels;
- decreased pharmacological complications and side effects.

Intrathecal drug delivery has been widely used for chronic malignant pain as well as chronic non-malignant pain since the 1980s, shortly after the discovery of opioid receptors in the central nervous system in the 1970s. In order to achieve the same therapeutic effect the intrathecal compartment only needs one-tenth of the epidural dose required and the epidural dose only needs one-tenth of the oral dose required. Thus the dose needed to achieve pain relief with intrathecal opioid administration is much less than an oral dose as the opioid is delivered directly to the site of action.

Current evidence shows that the use of intrathecal opioids is effective in reducing pain and increasing quality of life for chronic non-malignant pain such as pancreatitis, post-hepatic neuralgia and mixed pain states such as failed back surgery syndrome (FBSS) (Nitesuc et al., 1998), as well as chronic malignant pain (Gerber, 2003; Rauck et al., 2003).

Indications for intrathecal therapy

A trial of intrathecal opioids is indicated when:

- all other invasive and non-invasive treatment strategies have been tried and have failed to give adequate pain relief;
- the effect of oral opioids is inadequate due to intolerable side effects;
- life expectancy is greater than 6 months;
- psychological contraindications are excluded;
- the patient wishes to embark on long-term intrathecal therapy;
- the patient is able to understand the therapy and has adequate social support.

Intrathecal drug delivery can be used in the presence of nociceptive, neuropathic and mixed pains that have not achieved relief from simpler, less invasive treatment strategies.

Five phases of neuromodulation treatment

Patient selection and screening/physiological and psychological

It is important that an accurate diagnosis of the underlying pain aetiology and type is made before advanced neuromodulation is considered. Therefore thorough examination and history taking are vital.

Criteria to aid the selection process have gradually evolved over the many years that advanced neuromodulation has been in clinical use. These criteria include both physiological and psychological issues, and the performance of a trial screening period. Therefore the selection process for advanced neuromodulation is a multi-step process. Increased refinement of patient-selection criteria has been an important focus to improve advanced neuromodulation outcome, and, throughout the history of advanced neuromodulation application, there has been a search to refine patient selection criteria (Nelson et al., 1996). The goal of the selection process has developed in order to identify those patients for whom advanced neuromodulation will be most effective, while also assuring that resources are not expended unnecessarily.

Patients with chronic pain who are seen in a pain clinic have often already undergone numerous failures of treatment; yet another failure could be potentially damaging to the individual. Therefore the benefits of adequate patient selection are threefold:

- identifying those patients who are most likely to benefit from advanced neuromodulation;
- preventing unsuitable candidates from undergoing a costly invasive procedure;
- redirecting of unsuitable patients to more appropriate treatments.

The criteria are clearly defined in the EFIC European Consensus Statement (Gybels et al., 1998). The Consensus Statement highlights the importance of psychological screening and a clear diagnosis of the pain condition before proceeding to advanced neuromodulation implantation. In fact, in Belgium these criteria are essential for reimbursement.

Careful patient selection and screening offer the best chance of a positive outcome for advanced neuromodulation. Advanced neuromodulation should be considered when the following criteria are met:

- failed treatment with oral opioids or intolerable side effects (intrathecal therapy);
- life expectancy greater than 6 months (intrathecal therapy);
- failure of more conservative pain-management treatments;
- the patient is happy to consider a trial of the therapy;
- psychological assessment does not show any contraindications to advanced neuromodulation therapy.

Psychological exclusion criteria are:

- major psychiatric disorder;
- severe depression;
- somatization disorder;
- poor compliance, or lack of understanding about the procedure and treatment;
- lack of social support;
- drug or alcohol abuse;
- drug-seeking behaviour.

Many patients considered for advanced neuromodulation embark on a process of selection that often involves them in the decision-making process. In order to make an informed choice as to the appropriateness of advanced neuromodulation as a treatment for their pain, it is crucial that patients are armed with the relevant information. This would involve an educational input that addresses all aspects of SCS treatment including expectations of outcome and the possibility of treatment failure. This issue is of particular importance as these patients have often already undergone many treatment failures; in fact failure of other forms of pain relief including medication is primarily the reason why they are being considered for advanced neuromodulation.

Patient and family education

In order to make an informed choice the patient needs to be armed with the relevant information. Patient education for advanced neuromodulation should include all aspects of the therapy.

Referral to a SPD is often viewed as a last resort both by patients and by referring doctors. Patients can be apprehensive, fearful and hesitant about their upcoming advanced neuromodulation trial. They need to know that there is never a 100% guarantee that advanced neuromodulation will provide even partial relief. Successful outcomes are often related to expectations met. Therefore the primary goal of advanced neuromodulation patient education and preparation is to ensure the patient has realistic expectations regarding treatment outcome, particularly as a successful outcome is in no way guaranteed. Advanced neuromodulation involves patient participation not only during the procedure and the trial period but also with respect to ongoing pain management and rehabilitation.

Patients and their families or significant others need to be fully informed of the planned treatment and its practical consequences. It should be viewed as part of an active opt-in process. In order to make a decision the patient therefore has to be well informed as to the treatment itself, side effects, the trial, their own role in the therapy and long-term management. Patients are used to being viewed as passive receivers of care in the traditional medical model of cause and effect and they therefore act accordingly. Advanced neuromodulation therapy requires patients to be an active participant in their care. What may seem like a new approach to the patient needs to be carefully explained and reinforced. A passive patient who does not want to know about the therapy and just wants the doctor to get on with it would not be a good candidate for advanced neuromodulation. Usually a nurse specialist in pain management provides the education and preparation of the patient who is considering advanced neuromodulation. During this session, as well as discussing the practicalities of the therapy, a frank discussion of the patient's goals, expectations and responsibilities needs to be encouraged.

Trial of SCS and intrathecal delivery

Both advanced neuromodulation therapies require a trial-screening test to:

- assess the effectiveness of the intervention;

- observe the patient's response to pain relief;
- ensure appropriate use of the therapy.

Spinal cord stimulation (SCS) screening trial

The duration of the trial varies between pain centres. When assessing trial outcomes, patients are asked:

- Do they like the sensation?
- Do they achieve pain relief and to what degree?
- Are there any other improvements in quality of life, such as improved sleep quality?

If the trial is not successful the trial lead is removed. If the trial is successful then the whole SCS system is implanted. The patient can have a general anaesthetic for this procedure.

Intrathecal trial screening (IT)

An intrathecal drug trial can be performed either into the epidural space or the intrathecal space. The aim of the trial is to determine the patient's response to intrathecal opioids.

During the initial stages of an intrathecal trial the patient is kept in hospital to monitor side effects while the intrathecal opioid dose is titrated up and the oral dose of opioids is reduced. Once the dose is established patients can continue the trial at home allowing them the opportunity to judge the effects in their own environment. The average duration of an intrathecal trial is 4 weeks. Outcome of the trial screening is assessed in the chronic pain clinic. If the trial is unsuccessful the catheter is removed; if the trial is successful the catheter is still removed and a plan for implantation of a whole system is agreed with the patient.

Postoperative care

Spinal cord stimulation

Patients are monitored postoperatively during the trial period in order to:

- monitor for signs of infection;
- ensure adequate postoperative pain management;
- ensure patients understand how to operate the trial screener device;
- monitor and evaluate chronic pain relief and improvement in quality of life.

Intrathecal pump implant

During an intrathecal opioid trial the patient is kept in hospital until dose titration has been achieved and side effects either are not present or are managed appropriately. During this stage chronic pain is evaluated on a regular basis and the patient is encouraged to mobilize normally. The dose of opioid is gradually titrated up until satisfactory pain relief without side effects is achieved. Once this occurs the trial can continue in the patient's home. This allows patients to judge the pain relief when in their own environment.

Postoperatively the patient is monitored during the trial period in order to:

- monitor for signs of infection;
- ensure adequate postoperative pain management and management of any therapy-related side effects;
- ensure patients understand how to operate the external pump;
- monitor and evaluate chronic pain relief and improvement in quality of life.

Maintenance and long-term follow-up

Spinal cord stimulation

Long-term follow-up can involve reprogramming of the SCS device, encouragement regarding increasing activity and medication reduction advice. These patients are not discharged from the chronic pain service as they can require continued support and the SCS device may require maintenance.

Intrathecal pump

Once patients have an intrathecal pump implanted they will require regular visits to the chronic pain clinic to refill the pump. If they experience a sudden increase in their pain this could indicate a problem with the catheter or the pump. The patient needs to be able to access the pain team for trouble-shooting of the intrathecal system. Therefore, as with SCS patients, these patients cannot be discharged from the pain service and require continued long-term follow-up to ensure the safe delivery of intrathecal opioids and continuation of the therapy.

Conclusion

Chronic pain is a very complex phenonomen, which is not easy for healthcare professionals to treat or for the sufferer to manage and cope with. The search for a source or cause of the pain is important but when none can be found all those involved can become frustrated when restricted by the confines of the linear disease-centred medical model of care. Therefore chronic pain needs to be looked at from a more dynamic patient-centred holistic model of care, which uses the skills of many professions including psychology, nursing, medicine, occupational therapy and physiotherapy. If invasive procedures are used purely in isolation then it is less likely that the person in pain will gain any long-term benefit from the intervention. A chronic pain service needs to be able to access experienced pain specialists from health professions other than medicine.

Invasive pain-management procedures do have a place in the management of chronic pain but, as with all chronic pain treatment, including psychologically based interventions, they have limitations. These limitations are greater when a purely medical model of care is used. Patients need to be, and mostly want to be, involved in their treatment plan and every effort should be made to include them by providing good quality information and resources to ensure their expectations are realistic and can be met.

References

Aronoff GM, Evans WO, Enders PL (1983) A review of follow-up studies of multidisciplinary pain units. Pain 16: 1.

Bardense GAM, Weber W, Van Kleep M (1999) Treatment of spinal pain by means of radiofrequency procedures – part 1: the lumbar area. Pain Review 6: 143–53.

Boas RA (2002) Nerve blocks in chronic pain diagnosis. In Clinical Pain Management, Practical Applications and Procedures. Oxford: Oxford University Press.

Bogduk N, Lord SM (1998) Cervical zygapophyseal joint pain. Neurosurgery 8: 107–17.

Bonica JJ, Butler SH (1994) Local anaesthesia and regional blocks. In Wall PD, Melzack R (eds) Textbook of Pain, 3rd edn. Edinburgh: Churchill Livingstone.

Borg-Stein J, Stein, J (1996) Trigger points and tender points: one and the same? Does injection treatment help? Rheumatic Diseases Clinics of North America 22: 305–22.

Devor M, Govrin-Lippman R, Raber P (1985) Corticosteroids reduce neuroma hypersensitivity. In Fields HL, Dubner R, Cervero F (eds) Proceedings of the Fourth World Congress on Pain, Advances in Pain Research and Therapy, Vol. 9. New York: Raven Press, pp. 451–5.

Gerber HR (2003) Intrathecal morphine for chronic benign pain. Best practice and research. Clinical Anaesthesiology 17: 429–42.

Gybels J, Erdine S, Maeyeart J et al. (1998) Task Force of the European Federation of IASP Chapters EFIC Neuromodulation of Pain. A Consensus Statement. European Journal of Pain 2: 203–9.

Linderoff B, Foreman RD (1999) Physiology of spinal cord stimulation: review and update. Neuromodulation 2: 150–64.

Long DM (1991) Failed back surgery syndrome. Neurosurgery Clinics of North America 2: 899–919.

Mannheimer C, Eliasson T, Augustinsson LE et al. (1998) Electrical stimulation versus coronary artery bypass surgery in severe angina pectoris – the ESBY study. Circulation March: 1157–63.

Melzack R, Wall P (1965) Pain mechanisms. 'A new theory'. Science 150: 971–9.

Nelson DV, Kennington M, Novy DM et al. (1996) Psychological selection criteria for implantable spinal cord stimulation. Pain Forum 5: 93–103.

Nitesuc P, Dahm P, Applegren L, Currelaru I (1998) Continuous infusion of opioid and bupivacaine by externalised intrathecal catheters in long-term treatment of 'refractory nonmalignant pain'. Clinical Journal of Pain 14: 17–28.

North RB, Kidd DH, Lee MS, Piantodosi S (1994) A prospective, randomised study of spinal cord stimulation versus reoperation for failed back surgery syndrome Stereotactic and Functional Neurosurgery 62: 267–72.

Rauck RL, Cherry D, Boyer MF et al. (2003) Long-term intrathecal opioid therapy with a patient-activated, implanted delivery system for the treatment of refractory cancer pain. Journal of Pain 4: 441–7.

Simon DG, Travell LS, Simons LS (1999) Myofascial Pain and Dysfunction: The Trigger Point Manual, Vol 1, 2 edn. Baltimore, MD: Williams & Wilkins.

Simpson BA (1994) Spinal cord stimulation. Pain Reviews 1: 199–230.

Turner A, Loeser D, Kendra G (1995) Spinal cord stimulation for chronic low back pain: a systematic literature review. Neurosurgery 37: 1088–96.

Watts RW, Silagy A (1995) A meta-analysis of the efficacy of epidural corticosteroids in the treatment of sciatica. Anaesthesia and Intensive Care 23: 564–9.

CHAPTER SEVEN

Psychological perspectives

RUTH MADELEINE DALLOB, CRISTINA LÓPEZ-CHERTUDI
AND TRICIA ROSE

Aim

To provide general information about what psychology can offer to a pain-management service, specifying the role of the psychologist within a specialist pain team as well as how psychologists recognize when someone may need individual therapy.

Objectives

- To introduce the reader to the work of the psychologist and how it feels to work in an interdisciplinary team.
- To provide a view about the importance of team communication.
- To give the reader the knowledge to appreciate when referral to a pain-management programme could be ineffective and when individual therapy is needed.
- To offer the reader an appreciation of economic, social and occupational influences that may aggravate and/or perpetuate persistent pain cycles.

Introduction

Psychologists see people who deal with suffering and distress on a daily basis, bringing their personal stories, backgrounds, strengths and difficulties. Despite the universality of pain and suffering, pain still remains poorly understood: 'Pain is felt by all but it cannot be touched, seen or directly

155

measured, but its patterns can be recognised. Elusive and ill defined yet it has substance and specific characteristics' (Ch'u Ta Kao, 1985: 40).

'Pain upsets and destroys the nature of the person who feels it', the Greek philosopher Aristotle wrote (as cited in Ackrill, 1981). Following the passage of time, unrelieved pain creates physical, psychological and behavioural changes that reduce the quality of life. A recent shift in the recognition of pain and mental health issues has taken place, recognizing the importance of psychosocial processes. The limited success of purely physical interventions has led to a greater recognition of the importance of psychological processes.

Pain perception is a unique and very personal process. The people psychologists see are at different stages on their journey of acceptance of unexpected changes in their lives as a result of trauma, injury or pain. Family, employers, culture, beliefs, coping ability, expectations and past experiences all play an important part in the onset and maintenance of distress.

The relationship between distress and long-term pain

The chronic pain cycle

Pain is a multifaceted experience, an interaction of physiological, emotional, cognitive, sociocultural, behavioural and spiritual components. Pain perceptions and explanations about it vary from one individual to another and involve more than the painful physical sensation (Figure 7.1).

As touched on in Chapter 1, Melzack and Wall (1965) integrate sensory and psychological factors of the pain experience. One of the main implications of this model is that people's subjective experience of pain and their related behaviour may not be fully explained by physiological pathology alone, and psychological factors emerge as crucial in pain management. Lipton and Marbach (1984), Turk et al. (1992), Tota-Faucette et al. (1993) and Turk (1996, 1998), all explain the multiple dimensions of the pain experience by integrating psychological, sociocultural and physical factors.

Some clinicians assume that pathology or disease exists when pain is reported. Most people will have seen doctors and will have undergone various tests and procedures to try to identify pathology that matches their reported pain. Unfortunately, in many cases, by the time they have undergone these experiences, they may be feeling helpless and depressed because their pain has not as yet been 'cured' or they do not as yet have a 'label' for their pain condition.

If people believe they lack the resources to cope with persistent pain, they may feel vulnerable, become anxious in anticipation of harm and/or experience themselves as failing, which can lead to symptoms of anxiety or depression.

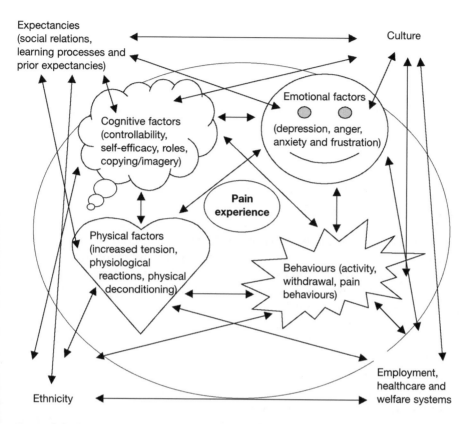

Figure 7.1 Complexity of chronic pain experience.

Perceptions of pain and mood (anger, depression and anxiety) are inter-related. While depression affects pain perception and the response of the individual to it, it also acts as a mediator between pain and disability. In order to avoid pain, disengagement from activities frequently occurs. If, however, the loss or costs incurred in avoiding an activity are too high then people will engage in the activity. This 'cost–benefit' ratio is most strongly influenced by the degree of depression experienced. As people become more avoidant they become more isolated and subsequently withdrawn.

A key factor in chronic pain is the belief that pain causes harm, which can predict disability (Waddell et al., 1984). A person with chronic pain may deteriorate from a fully functioning individual to someone who is inactive, spending long periods of time resting and taking pain medication that may have little or no effect. Some people search continually for treatments and the treatments continually fail (Maldonado, 1989).

Perceived physical disability may lead to a sense of loss of dignity, independence, employment or social status. When these potential threats become real, they may be seen as a permanent loss, which is then generalized to all aspects of personal worth and identity. The perception of personal disintegration may lead to symptoms and feelings of depression, which are interrelated with those of pain (Novy et al., 1995). In summary, chronic pain can lead to decreased activity, decreased levels of fitness and stamina, reduced self-esteem, hopelessness, social isolation and a decreased sense of control over pain (Turk and Holzman, 1986; Philips, 1988; Gatchel, 1991).

The economic and occupational context: the importance of work

The effect of pain is far reaching when it causes the person to be compromised in their ability to work; the emotional impact of this can be devastating. The impact will be extensive, affecting the individual's family, partners and friends, and most will suffer a loss of self-esteem as their perceived role within the family unit (if they are part of one) changes.

The response of individuals to pain is affected not only by their perception of the pain but also by their outlook regarding work and also possibly to entitlements to benefits if the original cause of pain was a work-related injury, or due to a trauma or an accident. The overall effects of pain and subsequent unemployment have crucial social effects.

Often people go to see a psychologist while still in the stages of seeking compensation, and with feelings of frustration or rage towards their employers. If they have been moved from their workplace due to the effects of their traumatic injury they may have associated feelings of sadness at losing colleagues and relationships as well as income.

When conducting psychological assessments, socioeconomic and occupational aspects of the person's life are explored in some depth in order to establish loss and also to identify any obstacles to recovery.

Hidden gains from pain

There can sometimes be 'hidden gains' within the overall pain experience. While the assistance from financial benefits provides protection in times of need in the event of prolonged absence from work, the individual may become reliant on financial support, which is payable only if a degree of incapacity remains. If people partially recover this may threaten their financial benefits without their knowing whether they may return to work or re-employment. This creates a difficult dilemma, especially if litigation is involved, as a return to their previous employment is less likely.

One of the most distressing aspects of ongoing litigation is that legal processes may take years to complete and people can be accused of exaggeration and malingering through the claim process. Any litigation case will need a physical and/or psychological examination; often several occur specifically for medico-legal purposes.

'Putting it on?'

Attribution of malingering as such is a legal matter to be dealt with in court, not for a medical expert (Mendelson, 1988). However, medical experts are requested to provide reports and comment on whether they think plaintiffs are exaggerating or faking their symptoms. While many clinicians consider their views to be expert 'some malingerers practice deception for a living, and can easily outmatch the physician who lacks the same type of experience, mental set and willingness for exploitation that sometimes characterises the professional con artist' (Faust, 1995).

There are some formal methods used to assess the person who is 'putting it on' (Main, 1999):

- diagnostic assessment according to psychiatric criteria;
- self-report measures designed to detect faking;
- symptom validity testing;
- elicitation of behavioural responses to examination;
- polygraphy.

Family and cultural influences

Cultural factors are not in themselves obstacles to recovery or rehabilitation but they can influence individuals differently. For example, people may hold different beliefs about the nature of pain and disability, depending on their cultural background.

It may be necessary to include the family in the assessment, as they can provide information about the person's way of relating to them, acceptance of shared goals for intervention as well as reliance or potential dependence on others and possible hidden gains from continual pain behaviour and resistance to change. It may be that a partner is upset or annoyed about the pain, or how it has been treated, or future treatment, and then the partner's response can affect the person in pain.

The impact of loss of role regarding work, either unpaid within the home or paid, will have an effect on the partner or other family members, who may have wanted to help, so preventing the person from attempting to change; or, conversely, the impact may be such that the individual feels rejected and unsupported.

Clarification of background information can be obtained through the assessment; possibly the individual's partner may have different perceptions and the process of dual interviewing can help clarify difficulties that may exist between couples and help assess the need for onward referral.

Psychological assessment

From the initial point of referral there often is a scheme whereby the person actively requests a consultation with the psychologist. This is known as the 'opt-in scheme', the aim being to promote a sense of control and active decision-making within the individual (see Appendix 1).

Preparing the individual for psychological assessment

People frequently arrive to see psychologists with a set of expectations, often along the lines of 'Am I seeing you because they think it's all in my head?'. This is addressed sensitively and a clear and honest explanation given that their experience of pain is genuine.

The purpose of a psychological assessment is:

- to assess the nature and type of pain to maximize long-term outcome;
- to explore overall stress and emotional status (two people with identical injuries may respond differently to treatment if one is severely anxious or depressed);
- to reassure about pain being real (not 'all in your mind');
- to explain the importance of physical and non-physical factors;
- to give recommendations and feedback after assessment.

The aim of the assessment is to try to determine to what extent psychological factors such as depression, financial difficulties, loss of usual work and domestic role, relationship problems and social withdrawal affect the person. A full explanation about the purpose of the assessment, its length and aspects of confidentiality will help to relieve the anxiety of seeing a psychologist for the first time.

The psychological assessment can be carried out using a semi-structured interview format. It actively involves the person and explores options to address all components of pain. The psychological assessment:

- explores psychological factors to be addressed in treatment (unhelpful beliefs, secondary gains);
- suggests treatments that may help resolve psychological risk factors;

- ascertains appropriateness of pain treatments according to individual needs;
- provides clues on how someone may respond to treatment;
- identifies people most likely to benefit from the proposed interventions (either neuromodulation, pain-management programmes or individual therapy);
- plans a comprehensive intervention based on the multidimensionality of pain.

The assessment needs to evaluate:

- effectiveness of previous strategies used to relieve pain (physiotherapy, hydrotherapy, counterstimulation or others);
- participants' beliefs about their pain condition/coping ability/impact on overall lifestyle;
- factors exacerbating or maintaining pain symptoms;
- previous relevant history to provide information about vulnerability to developing psychological difficulties in stressful situations;
- stability of current environment (drug or alcohol use, severe stressors from family, social or work environments, sources of income, ongoing compensation cases);
- willingness to participate in and commitment to engage with treatment;
- short-term goals;
- current psychological state.

In summary, a thorough psychological assessment can help us understand the predisposing, enabling and reinforcing factors that affect chronic pain.

After assessment, what next?

The outcome of the assessment may comprise four main options: individual sessions offered at the pain clinic, onward referral to a more appropriate service, case conferences or team discussions, and attendance at a pain-management programme. These options are discussed in detail below.

Reasons for providing individual therapy

During the assessment, potential risk factors such as suicidal ideation, suicide attempts or self-harming behaviours are identified. Other factors are the extent to which psychological difficulties impinge on the mental well-being of the person, in that the individual could not function within a group, is at risk or could be disruptive to the group process (as explained below). This may be because of either aggressive behaviour or fearfulness in a group setting. A set of inclusion/exclusion criteria is followed (see Appendix 2), which is used as a tool to help differentiate who would be most helped by a choice of either individual or group intervention.

The psychologist who undertakes the assessment may be the best person to offer individual therapy, as a rapport will be established from the initial consultation. A number of one-to-one sessions are agreed, with a clear objective. Individual sessions then occur in the same way as therapy would in any clinic setting, with a clear agreed contract. Assessment is flexible and ongoing, a process rather than a one-off meeting.

Unresolved grief and previous physical or sexual abuse are fairly common psychological problems, which may impinge on functioning. Deeper exploration of these issues could make the individual better prepared to subsequently attend a group, able to absorb the educational aspects and respond to the ideas introduced in the group programme. However, this will depend entirely on the individual and, even after therapy, the person may not fulfil the criteria for attending the pain-management programme and they may need onward referral to other services.

Other reasons for offering individual therapy would include the need to prepare the individual for working with others in a group. People may be so overwhelmed at discovering that there is no 'active cure' for their chronic pain that they need time to work through their feelings, which often include grief at the loss of hope for a cure. They may need time to accept the need to consider ways of adjusting to living with their pain.

Some reasons people may not initially be considered for a pain-management programme may include an inability to function within a group due to their overwhelming feelings of anger or grief, related to loss, or loss of role or difficulties in relationships. Their personalities may be such that they are overwhelmed by shyness and cannot imagine speaking in front of others.

An assessment is made as to whether individual sessions beforehand will have a positive impact before group treatment will be offered. Often, the one-to-one sessions will be sufficiently therapeutic, so that the individual goes on to develop further and then be offered the opportunity to attend the pain-management programme.

Onward referral

There may be situations where the psychologist may not offer therapy but where onward referral to a specialist agency is more appropriate. This may include, for example, where there is substance misuse. If people wish to alter their behaviour they can be given information about self-referral to an appropriate agency so that issues of substance misuse can be addressed.

Any major psychological difficulties need to be identified at assessment or through information provided by other mental healthcare professionals prior to assessment. These difficulties need to be addressed by appropriate services such as psychiatric services or community mental health teams.

It has been estimated that a significant proportion of people referred to pain-management services suffer an identifiable psychiatric illness (Main and Spanswick, 2000). These include anxiety disorders, post-traumatic stress disorder, clinical depression, somatoform disorders, hypochondriasis, adjustment disorders and personality disorders.

If the psychologists in the pain team are unaware of any psychiatric problems, these may become apparent through the process of the thorough and extensive assessment. One of the reasons for the lengthy assessment is the need to detect these difficulties, which may have been hidden up to this point.

Case conferences or team discussions and their value

People with complex difficulties need the input from each member of the team as they all have a unique contribution to make. After an assessment from each member the team would meet together to discuss the best way forward. It may be that the individual is not ready to embark on the pain-management programme, or there is concern about, for example, expectations regarding neuromodulation therapy.

It is often necessary to instigate team meetings with all the key members of the team who are involved in this person's care, inviting him or her and the partner or spouse to attend so they are actively involved in these discussions, decisions and outcomes. The 'patient' thus becomes a person, by using a philosophy of self-empowerment and non-directive interventions to enable own decisions and own goals to be reached.

Pain-management programme

Who runs a PMP?

A pain-management programme (PMP) is intradisciplinary. Each member of this integrated team has learned and borrowed knowledge from the other professions forming the team to give a unified and consistent message. There is a strong overlap between the various professions that constitute the team (consultant in anaesthesia and pain management, clinical/counselling psychologists, nurse specialist in pain, physiotherapist and occupational therapist). They are experienced in their fields and have received the relevant training and ongoing supervision.

What does the psychologist do in a PMP?

Superficially, the role of psychologists on a PMP may not be as obvious as the roles of the other health professions: medicine, nursing and physio-therapy. Psychologists work with emotions, thought processes and behaviour. So what is their relevance in a pain-management team? This is often an initial concern of the people attending a PMP: 'aha, so you do think the pain is all in my head!' or 'so you think I'm mad!'. The psychologist aims to enable people to take control of their pain and of their own pain-management skills. By giving them back control, the psychologist hopes to improve their ability to cope with the pain.

There are two key areas of involvement for psychologists.

The first is psychoeducational:

- education about how pain is perceived and the interplay of emotions, thought processes, imagery and pain;
- dealing with the practicalities of pain and providing people with management techniques;
- discussing issues that might arise alongside the pain, such as sleep and sexual problems or communication difficulties.

The second is therapeutic:

- Assessing and preparing potential participants before the programme. This is an opt-in programme – nobody is obliged to attend. Even from the initial stages, psychologists are promoting a sense of personal control. It is important that the people on the programme are motivated (it can be hard work, people will get out what they put in and spaces are limited and costly) and have sufficient capacity for understanding, self-awareness and self-reflection.
- Dealing with mental health issues during the programme. There is a high co-occurrence of depression and chronic pain (Magni et al., 1993, 1994; Rajala et al., 1995; Turk et al., 1995; McCracken, 1996). Anxiety coincides with chronic pain when anticipation of the pain occurs (Philips, 1988; Arntz et al., 1994).
- Monitoring and managing group dynamics. Although this type of intervention has a strong educational component, it is still a therapeutic one – there is more emotional interplay and it promotes change, self-awareness and personal growth. For example, significant levels of anxiety, anger, depression or a sense of loss may be experienced. Specific mem-

bers of the group may feel hostile towards health professionals whom they perceive as having failed them.

Sometimes the programme may be the participant's first chance to talk with other people who are suffering with chronic pain. This can be a very positive support group experience. However, it can also cause difficulties for some people who perhaps may feel their pain is 'not as severe as everyone else's' or is 'different from' that of others.

The role of the psychologists is to try to monitor these processes, enhancing the positive aspects and minimizing disruptive elements. In order to facilitate group members' participation the psychologist works towards enabling change within the individual. Basic tasks are to show concern, acceptance, genuineness and empathy, which in turn may facilitate the creation, maintenance and shaping of the group into a therapeutic social system. During the programme, difficult and personal issues can be discussed, and people may find their mood affected by these. So, the psychologist also tries to maintain a safe, supportive environment and to be available for individual discussions if necessary.

- Discussing with the rest of the team the potential psychological issues as they arise and learning from the other members of the team.

What does a PMP include?

The PMP can be an outpatient or inpatient group intervention, using a multidisciplinary approach based on cognitive–behavioural and systemic principles and methods to manage chronic pain. It aims to help individuals improve their quality of life, despite the pain, by gaining greater control. This is an integrative and holistic programme that aims to address both emotional and physical aspects of pain, without offering a total cure for it.

The PMP involves education. Pain experience is introduced as a universal, individual and complex experience within a biopsychosocial and spiritual framework. The gate-control theory of pain is reviewed to clarify the connections among emotions, thinking processes, imagery and perception of pain levels. People gain an understanding of what factors modulate this gate mechanism.

The multifaceted nature of pain (physiological, emotional, cognitive, social, cultural, spiritual) is reviewed and the impact on people's lives explored (Figure 7.2).

Participants are asked to identify unhelpful and unrealistic thoughts and beliefs associated with pain and emotional distress (such as anger, frustration, depression or anxiety). They are encouraged to modify those related to reduced self-esteem, catastrophizing, fear avoidance, high standards, and loss of control affecting their responses to pain.

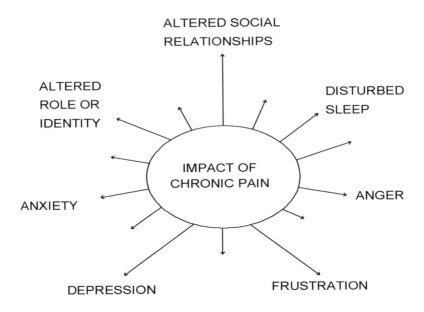

Figure 7.2 The multifaceted nature of pain. The dynamic interaction between these factors is recognized with the aim of breaking unhelpful vicious cycles.

Participants are encouraged to self-reflect and to monitor their emotional distress and thought processes in a given situation. Finally, they consider more helpful thoughts focusing on a greater sense of personal control and self-reliance. For example, they may monitor their anticipation of pain, which may lead to feelings of apprehension and anxiety; they may then start doubting their ability to cope with pain. By practising abdominal breathing or relaxation, they may manage to minimize tension and anxiety, which may give a greater sense of confidence in their control over pain.

Thought-stopping techniques and the use of coping statements are encouraged. Participants are also encouraged to monitor and break the various 'vicious cycles' (overactivity/underactivity) by decreasing overt pain behaviour through negative reinforcement and/or increasing well behaviour by positive reinforcement.

The physiological and psychological effects of the relaxation response are reviewed. Breathing and passive muscle relaxation techniques, as well as guided imagery, are taught. Distraction techniques are also taught to divert participants' focus on pain (Fishman, 1992). Participants are encouraged to practise relaxation at home and to monitor their performance.

Disturbed sleep can be managed by promoting 'sleep hygiene' techniques (retraining sleep patterns, creating a stimulus-free environment), relaxation and improved posture.

Gentle and graduated exercise and stretching are used to improve fitness and flexibility, to build up muscle strength and stamina through activity and, finally, to re-educate posture and movement. Participants record their performance in time-limited exercises based on activities of daily living to monitor their improvement each week. Their performance on certain activities may be videotaped at the beginning and end of the intervention. Talks on self-massage, heat/cold treatment, structure of the spine, ergonomics and body mechanics are given.

A PMP includes goal setting and pacing. The principles of activity pacing are explained and participants are encouraged to break down tasks into gradual stages and to plan regular and manageable levels of activity, monitoring whether their pattern of activity is contributing to increased pain. Participants are encouraged to set either short-term or long-term goals in the areas of work, leisure activities, social life and domestic tasks, which are jointly considered by the participants and the team to be attainable. Individual baselines and rate of achievements are monitored. The team, other members of the programme and the video feedback session provide reinforcement of achievements.

Medication management can be addressed in a PMP. Education can be provided about pain-related drugs, tranquillizers, sedatives and antidepressants. Medication intake is reviewed with each participant and an individual management plan is agreed aiming to reduce medication that has not proved helpful in improving the participant's pain or function.

A PMP can contribute to an improvement in communication skills. It can provide advice on different ways of communicating with family, friends, social and work circles, as well as health professionals, about living with pain and changes in roles. Assertiveness and anger management skills are taught and practised. By identifying potential areas of difficulty, allowing people to discuss these and suggesting some ways of improving communication, people learn to express their needs more clearly and more assertively. Unhelpful pain behaviours are identified and challenged. Issues regarding intimate relations are also discussed in a safe and confidential environment.

Coping, self-efficacy and perceived control can be addressed. These skills and strategies contribute to people developing a sense of control over pain by increasing their confidence in their ability to gain mastery and self-esteem, reducing the stresses associated with pain and its consequences (loss of role and employment, relationship difficulties, sense of loss of dignity) and adopting self-regulating coping strategies.

Relaxation training for the management of chronic pain

There are a number of well-defined relaxation interventions, some of which are commonly used to treat chronic pain. Research supports the effectiveness of relaxation as a method of persistent pain management. One study compared the effectiveness of relaxation, exercise and a combination of the two, with people suffering from fibromyalgia. It was found that all three treatment groups produced improvements in self-efficacy for physical function, which was best maintained by the combination group after a 2-year follow-up period (Buckelew et al., 1998, cited in Sultanoff and Zalaquett, 2000).

Benson (1975, 1983, cited in Sultanoff and Zalaquett, 2000) argued that all relaxation techniques produce a single state; he termed this the 'relaxation response', characterized by diminished sympathetic arousal. The autonomic nervous system has two branches: the sympathetic and the parasympathetic. The state of deep relaxation stimulates the parasympathetic nervous system, which promotes calmness. The state produced by the exact opposite of the parasympathetic nervous system is commonly termed the 'fight or flight' response. In this response the sympathetic branch of the autonomic nervous system is aroused, producing emotional and physiological reactions that can be activated at times of emergency, thus allowing the body to 'fight or flee'. This is a normal and necessary response to danger. Some of the changes that occur when the mind and body are in a state of deep relaxation are given below (the list is adapted from Benson (1975, cited in Bourne, 1995):

- decrease in heart rate;
- decrease in respiration rate;
- decrease in blood pressure;
- decrease in skeletal muscle tension;
- decrease in metabolic rate and muscle tension;
- increase in skin resistance;
- increase in alpha-wave activity in the brain;
- increased energy levels;
- improved concentration and memory;
- reduction of insomnia and fatigue;
- increased self-confidence and reduced self-blame;
- increased availability of feelings;
- decrease in analytical thinking.

The exact opposite of the above psychophysiological state is produced by the activation of the sympathetic branch of the autonomic nervous system.

Schwartz, Davidson and Goleman (1978, cited in Sultanoff and

Zalaquett, 2000) suggested that the majority of relaxation procedures have highly specific effects, as well as more general stress-reducing effects; therefore, the specific effects of various relaxation techniques may be superimposed upon a general relaxation effect. For example, both diaphragmatic breathing and progressive muscle relaxation can be used for specific effect, slowing the breathing and relaxing the muscles. However, both can produce a general state of relaxation.

Relaxation methods

There are a vast number of relaxation methods. The methods briefly mentioned here are those that have found to be effective in the management of chronic pain. Diaphragmatic breathing, guided imagery, progressive muscle relaxation and autogenic training have extensive literatures in their own right. The use of music is a personal choice; it can act as either a distraction from pain or an enhancement of the relaxation response.

Breathing (diaphragmatic)

When teaching relaxation training, we talk about the 'art of breathing'. Diaphragmatic breathing is the healthiest form of breathing; it is fundamental with most relaxation methods. It is also the most natural; observe how young babies breathe; they will use their diaphragm and full torso for each breath. As adults we tend to lose the 'art of breathing' and habitually breathe from the upper chest. Although not wrong, upper-chest breathing will be shallow and more rapid (in a waking state) than if you were using your diaphragm. Upper-chest breathing does not allow the upper ribcage to expand and contract; therefore, the amount you inhale and exhale is considerably less.

Imagery

Achterberg (1985, as cited in Sultanoff and Zalaquett, 2000) defined imagery as mental processes that summon and use the five senses: vision, audition, smell, taste and touch.

Guided imagery is the process of using narration and sometimes music, to take the listeners on an inner journey to scenic and peaceful places. The trainer invites the listeners to use all five senses to image the journey, prompting for colour, smell and texture. The more vivid the image the more real it can feel. Imagery can also be used in a more focused form; for example; the image of a dial or switch to regulate pain intensity, or ice for a burning sensation and warmth for muscle tension. Many responses in the body do not distinguish between having a physical experience and imagining having that experience. It has been argued that imagery has limitations regarding reducing somatic symptoms and muscle tension. People with chronic pain may be unable to create images due to pain intensity. It is therefore important to combine it with breathing methods and/or progressive muscle relaxation.

Progressive muscle relaxation

Edmund Jacobson developed the progressive muscle relaxation model in the late 1930s. The basic idea is to isolate each muscle group systematically and practise tensing and relaxing the groups of muscles. The process of progressive muscle relaxation is simply to create tension for 8–10 seconds, and then let the muscle relax and the tension go.

Once the muscles relax then other components of the relaxation response will naturally follow. Relaxed muscles require less oxygen so breathing slows and deepens. Heart rate and blood pressure decline and the body begins to feel warm. Within the remit of persistent pain management, progressive muscle relaxation is adapted into two methods. Active muscle relaxation requires clenching and then releasing the muscles. Passive muscle relaxation requires *imagining* the tension in the muscles and then releasing. This can be helpful when pain and stiffness make clenching difficult and can also prevent the occurrence of muscle spasms.

Autogenics

Autogenics is the name given to a relaxation technique developed by Schultz and Luthe in the 1920s. The term means generated from within. The basic idea is that the body should follow the dictates of the mind. It consists of a series of statements you repeat to yourself. The emphasis is on warmth and heaviness, for example: *My arm is warm . . . My arm is heavy . . . My arm is warm and heavy.* These simple statements have a cumulative effect and allow the body to sink into a deep state of relaxation. As with diaphragmatic breathing and progressive muscle relaxation, autogenic relaxation decreases the heart rate and blood pressure, the limbs become heavy and the body warms up. Empirical evidence has shown that autogenic relaxation has helped in the treatment of insomnia, headaches and chronic pain.

The environment

A safe, calm and comfortable environment is essential for the practice of relaxation if it is to be successful. There should be no disturbances from children, neighbours, telephones, pagers or tradesmen. Hang a notice on the door if necessary. A reclining chair, mat or cushions will give the body support. When the relaxation response is induced, the body temperature drops, so make sure there is a blanket at hand or that the room is comfortably warm. The ability to master relaxation will depend on the time given. It needs to be practised on a daily basis. Make it a part of life and do not use the 'time myth' ('I don't have time').

Although relaxation can help reduce the effects of stress and anxiety, a person in a state of high anxiety, deep distress or high agitation (all of which can occur with the presence of chronic pain) would find it extremely difficult to obtain a state of relaxation. Sadigh (2001: 66) lists the psychological conditions that are better managed in conjunction with the psychology and/or the psychiatric services:

- severe anxiety;
- major depressive illness;
- active psychosis;
- severe manic episode;
- dissociative identity disorder (during active phrase);
- severe distress following a trauma;
- thought disorder due to psychological or organic causes.

Inexperienced relaxation trainers should not consider relaxation training with any persons exhibiting the above conditions. Within the realm of the chronic pain service, psychological screening would identify these disorders.

Summary of PMP participant feedback

This is a summary of accounts about coping strategies people were using after having attended a PMP, which gives us an idea of what aspects of the PMP people found most useful. According to the participants, the most frequently reported coping strategy after treatment was related to cognitive factors. Some participants stated that they were more able to adopt more constructive thought processes. Some reported being more able to accept their chronic pain condition and the resulting limitations in function or role. For others, education about pain-related aspects contributed to their understanding of pain and, consequently, this knowledge enabled them to cope better with the pain.

The individuals' coping skills were diverse. Many of the coping strategies taught in the PMP were being used by participants after treatment. In some cases the psychoeducational approach (explanation of gate-control theory of pain and the multifaceted dimension of pain) may have contributed to normalizing their distress. For some, understanding the connection between pain and thinking could be a way of empowering them with a sense of self-centredness and underlying self-confidence. This may be linked to those cognitive techniques that promoted self-monitoring to identify underlying unrealistic thought processes and assumptions about their perceived loss of control, which affect responses to pain.

Some participants also reported an improvement in mood. They reported that mental distraction and relaxation techniques helped them to control their pain. Moreover, goal setting and problem solving were reported to be beneficial in the areas of work, leisure, and social and domestic activities.

In the physical/behavioural areas, some used pacing of activities and relaxation to achieve goals. Certain participants also reported an improvement in sleep pattern, a reduction in pain-related behaviours and a reduction of unhelpful medication.

Some stated that communication channels between themselves and a circle of friends and relatives had improved. As mentioned above, it is essential to consider the effect that chronic pain has on people perceiving themselves as socially isolated. Their psychological distress (depression, anxiety or frustration) may be affecting the family dynamics or other significant relations. This social dimension could be related to communication in the group setting. Participants found support from the staff and other members of the group.

Some participants stated that they had managed to improve their lifestyles by developing new hobbies or interests and by engaging more in daily activities.

Some people returned to work, after a prolonged period of being on benefits; a small proportion declined the option of spinal surgery and returned to college to learn new skills; one person received a much-wanted promotion; others returned to adult education to retrain. Some of these people are of an age where re-employment is unlikely.

Overall, participants reported skills such as more constructive thinking styles and new behavioural patterns brought about by using exercise, stretching, relaxation, pacing and goal setting. For some, these skills resulted in the perceived promotion of personal control over pain (increased self-confidence and self-centredness).

Team communication

Within a 'good' team, each member is aware of the roles of the others. This is crucially important as otherwise care that could be offered is neglected. Some teams can work individually in the delivery of care for months without being aware of what others can offer or how to refer to each other.

The key features of the interdisciplinary team can be summarized as:

- The team members all share common assessment and treatment goals.
- The main task of all team members is to deliver treatments that are based on the needs of the individual, not the constraints of the individual professionals involved.
- Unlike multidisciplinary teams, a member of the medical profession may not lead interdisciplinary teams. They can be led by an experienced clinician who has knowledge of working with people in chronic pain and also of working in a team.
- There are core areas of speciality related to each discipline but these take second place to the goals of the team as a whole. All the team members have explicit knowledge of the skills of other members in the team.
- Communication occurs between all team members.
- Decisions are made after considering input from all team members.

In contrast, multidisciplinary teams tend to be:

- led by a member of the medical profession, in which formal communication occurs and members 'report back' in a hierarchical fashion to the team leader;
- limited to the skills and knowledge of the team member's own discipline (Main and Spanswick, 2000).

For teams to work effectively, each member needs to have a healthy respect for what each team member brings to provide the most effective care. Professionals each see the person from a different perspective but have an area of care that is their main focus, with overlapping skills relating to many other aspects. For example, the nurse specialist in pain management may have expertise in medication and dry needling but also has advanced communication and psychological skills and it is perhaps this aspect that overlaps considerably with all the team members.

Achieving success in treatment

Success in dealing with chronic pain does not mean completely eliminating it. Treatment can be considered successful if people feel in control and able to manage their difficulties. Tools to manage pain and techniques for improving quality of life have been offered. Following individual therapy or the PMP individuals may have worked through their psychological difficulties, for example problems in relationships, expressed their feelings and achieved new perspectives of viewing the problem, and then set goals after deciding to manage the situation differently.

The tools of reframing unhelpful beliefs and applying them to difficult situations will have been given and hopefully used. Outcomes can be evaluated with questionnaires following national guidelines, but perhaps the richest source of data is the self-report where the person evaluates change and effectiveness.

Implications

The overall aim of offering psychological perspectives when managing chronic pain is that people change their view from that of pain being the result of a failed medical procedure and begin to understand that their pain may never go away completely, but that they can have some control to minimize the impact of pain in their lives. Both through the group process within the PMP and through individual therapy, the person may be helped when recognizing that others may be more badly affected physically, that there are alternative ways of coping and that each response to pain and suffering is unique and special to the individual.

Understanding pain as a subjective experience (Fernandez and Turk, 1992: 205) validates the person's private inner reality. However, when the reality and genuineness of pain are questioned as being 'psychological' in nature, people feel invalidated because pain is not accessible to the outside world.

People normally express their difficulty recognizing the psychological factors in pain perception, as their understanding of pain is based on a biomedical perspective and most people are seeking a cure. Current services are based on Western medical approaches within which pain is viewed as an enemy to be conquered and treatments are weapons to use against this enemy (Notcutt, 1998).

Psychology has been viewed in medical settings as an add-on profession. A change of culture within professional settings has been required. Teams and disciplines at pain clinics are starting to embrace the biopsychosocial model more willingly.

People normally see psychologists as expert professionals, making us even more aware of our own vulnerabilities, limitations and mortality.

Conclusion

The potential integration of psychological and sociocultural domains with physical factors within a biopsychosocial and spiritual framework has been examined as a way of understanding chronic pain, disability and related psychological distress.

The psychological effects of long-term pain are lasting and interfere with vocational, interpersonal, domestic areas and physical health. Appraisal, personality, emotional states, coping skills, social support and compensation status are important psychosocial factors when conceptualizing and planning interventions for chronic pain. Moreover, successful interventions require an individualized and flexible approach that takes into account some of the wider issues of our clinical practice.

Several psychological approaches can be combined. The clinician needs to identify the sources of distress and how they are accessible to treatment, perhaps making decisions about how one level of impairment interferes when trying to address other levels. The psychologist and the person in pain walk along the path together, aware of a general direction but also open to new discoveries.

References

Ackrill JL (1981) Aristotle the Philosopher. Oxford: Oxford University Press.

Arntz A, Dreessen L, De Jong P (1994) The influence of anxiety on pain: attentional and attributional mediators. Pain 56: 307–14.

Bourne E (1995) The Anxiety and Phobia Workbook. Oakland, CA: New Harbinger Publications.

Ch'u Ta Kao (1985) Tao Te Ching. London: Unwin.

Doleys DM, Klapow JC, Hammer M (1997) Psychological evaluation in spinal cord stimulation therapy. Pain Reviews 4: 189–207.

Faust D (1995) The detection of deception. In Weintraub MI (ed.) Neurological Clinics, Vol 13(2) Malingering and Conversion Reactions. Philadelphia, PA: WB Saunders.

Fernandez E, Turk DC (1992) Sensory and affective components of pain: separation and synthesis. Psychological Bulletin 112: 205–17.

Fishman B (1992) The cognitive-behavioural perspective on pain management in terminal illness. Hospital Journal 8(1–2): 73–88.

Gatchel RJ (1991) Early development of physical and mental deconditioning in painful spinal disorders. In Mayer TG, Mooney V, Gatchel RJ (eds) Contemporary Conservative Care for Painful Spinal Disorders. Philadelphia: Lea & Febiger, pp. 278–89.

Lipton JA, Marbach JJ (1984) Ethnicity and the pain experience. Social Science and Medicine 19: 1279–98.

Lusk JT (1993) (ed.) Thirty Scripts for Relaxation, Imagery and Inner Healing. Duluth, MN: Whole Persons Associates Inc.

McCracken LM (1991) Cognitive-behavioral treatment of rheumatoid arthritis: a preliminary review of efficacy and methodology. Annals of Behavioral Medicine 13(2): 57–65.

McCracken LM, Gross RT, Aikens J et al. (1996) The assessment of anxiety and fear in persons with chronic pain: a comparison of instruments. Behavioural Research and Therapy 34: 927–33.

Main CJ (1999) Medico-legal aspects of pain: the nature of psychological opinion in cases of personal injury. In Gatchel RJ, Turk DC (eds) Psychological Factors of Pain. New York: Guilford Press, pp 132–47.

Main CJ, Spanswick CC (2000) Pain Management, An Interdisciplinary Approach. London: Churchill Livingstone.

Magni G, Marchetti M, Moreschi C et al. (1993) Chronic musculoskeletal pain and depressive symptoms in the national health and nutrition examination I. Epidemiologic follow-up study. Pain 53: 163–8.

Magni G, Moreschi C, Rigatti-Luchini S et al. (1994) Prospective study on the relationship between depressive symptoms and chronic musculoskeletal pain. Pain 56: 289–97.

Maldonado L (1989) Behavioral concepts, methods and approaches to pain management. Psychotherapy in Private Practice 7(4): 17–29.

Melzack R, Wall PD (1965) Pain mechanisms: a new theory. Science 150: 971–9.

Mendelson G (1988) Psychiatric Aspects of Personal Injury Claims. Springfield, IL: Charles C Thomas.

Notcutt W (1998) The Tao of pain. Pain Reviews 5: 203–15.

Novy DM, Nelson DV, Berry LA et al. (1995) What does the Beck Depression Inventory measure in chronic pain? A re-appraisal. Pain 61: 261–70.

Philips HC (1988) The Psychological Management of Chronic Pain: A Treatment Manual. New York: Springer.

Rajala U, Keinanen-Kiukaanniemi S, Uusimaki A, Kivela SL (1995) Musculoskeletal pains and depression in a middle-aged Finnish population. Pain 61: 451–7.

Sadigh MR (2001) Autogenic Training: A Mind and Body Approach to the Treatment of Fibromyalgia and Chronic Pain Syndrome. New York: The Haworth Medical Press, p. 65.

Sultanoff B, Zalaquett C (2000) Relaxation therapies. In Novey DW (ed.) Clinician's Complete Reference to Complementary and Alternative Medicine. New York: Mosby, pp. 114–29.

Tota-Faucette ME, Gil KM, Williams FJ, Goli V (1993) Predictors of response to pain management treatment: the role of family environment and changes in cognitive processes. Clinical Journal of Pain 9: 115–23.

Turk DC (1996) Biopsychosocial perspective on chronic pain. In Gatchel RJ, Turk DC (eds) Psychological Approaches to Pain Management. New York: Guilford Publications Inc.

Turk DC (1998) Biopsychosocial perspective on chronic pain. In Block AR, Kremer EF (eds) Handbook of Pain Syndromes: Biopsychosocial Perspectives, Conceptual and Diagnostic Issues. New York: Lawrence Erlbaum Associates Inc., pp. 3–32.

Turk DC, Holzman AD (1986) Chronic pain: interface among physical, psychological and social parameters. In Holzman AD, Turk DC (eds) Pain Management: A Handbook of Psychological Approaches. New York: Pergamon, pp. 1–19.

Turk DC, Kerns RD, Rosenberg R (1992) Effects of marital interaction on chronic pain and disability: examining the down-side of social support. Rehabilitation Psychology 37: 259–74.

Turk DC, Okifuji A, Scharff L (1995) Chronic pain and depression: role of perceived impact and perceived control in different age cohorts. Pain 61: 93–101.

Waddell G, Main CJ, Morris EW et al. (1984) Chronic low-back pain, psychologic distress, and illness behavior. Spine 9: 209–13.

Wilson KG, Mikail SF, D'Eon JL et al. (1993) Depression in the context of pain: a survey of IASP members. Paper presented at the Seventh World Congress on Pain, Paris, France.

Appendix 1: pain-management service referral opt-in system

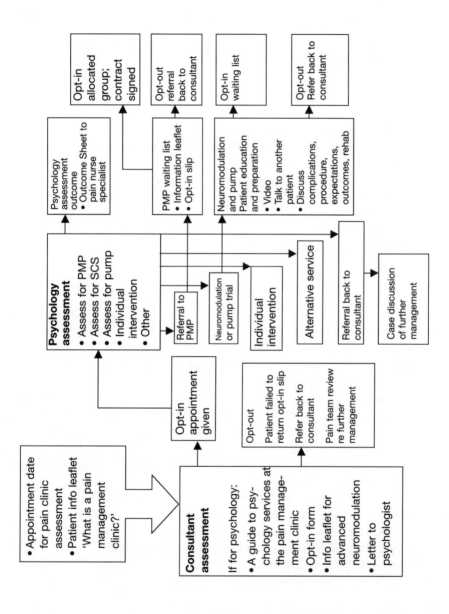

Appendix 2: PMP inclusion/exclusion criteria

Inclusion

- Experiencing pain for more than 6 months.
- Wishing to participate in the group and formally opting in by signing a contract of attendance.
- Presenting at least one of the following as a result of experiencing long-term pain:
  - widespread disruption of activity/functioning;
  - overactivity and/or underactivity;
  - excessive or inappropriate medication use;
  - use of unnecessary aids;
  - excessive pain behaviours (guarding posture, inactivity, grimace);
  - work reduced or impaired;
  - emotional distress (anger, anxiety, depression, stress);
  - unhelpful attitudes/pain perception;
  - unhelpful communication styles;
  - self-reported difficulties in interpersonal relations (unassertive, passive, aggressive);
  - reduced self-confidence/esteem.

Exclusion

- Age below 16 years.
- Declining to opt-in.
- Actively receiving or seeking medical or psychological treatment for long-term pain elsewhere.
- Potential to be disruptive to the group process (based on the team's clinical opinion and/or client's reported range of antisocial, social-phobic, aggressive behaviour or fearfulness of participation in a group setting).
- A severe disability due to impairment other than due to long-term pain (for example, blind and deaf, unable to lip-read) unless alternative provisions can be made.
- A severe psychological disorder, which is better addressed prior to the PMP (for example, severe post-traumatic stress disorder).
- Lacking full use of spoken and written English.
- Being unavailable for the duration of the programme.
- Showing substance misuse.
- Being actively psychotic and/or actively suicidal.

Note: these criteria need to be flexible and based on sound clinical judgement.

Appendix 3: relaxation scripts

Breathing (diaphragmatic)

Test your breathing using the method below.

- Rest one hand on your upper chest and the other over your tummy.
- Notice which hand rises first when you inhale.
- If the upper hand rises first you are using upper chest breathing. If the lower hand rises first you are breathing with your diaphragm. If both move at the same time you are using a mix of both.

Exercise

- Lie flat on the floor or sit in a chair. Make sure that you are fully supported.
- Put one palm on your upper chest and the other over your abdomen. (The objective is to have the hand on the abdomen rise first when you breathe in.)
- Breathe out fully – and then a little bit more. With practice you will find you can do this by drawing in your abdomen. Pause for 4 seconds.
- Allow the air to flow in naturally again.
- Repeat this cycle a few times.

[Practise this for a few minutes on a daily basis. When teaching this exercise it is important to observe the movement of the hands. If the person seems to be having difficulty, it would be helpful to model the correct positioning of the hands.]

Make sure that you are comfortable, arms and legs uncrossed. Now become aware of your breathing, focus on your breathing, hear and sense every breath you take. Breathe in through your nose, be aware of the breath entering your nostrils, and be aware of the breath being exhaled from your mouth.

Lay one hand on your chest and the other below your chest resting on your abdomen.

Imagine that you have a balloon inside your abdomen. As you inhale the balloon inflates; inhale until you can imagine that the balloon fills the abdomen.

Now exhale slowly through your mouth; keep exhaling until you can imagine that the balloon is fully deflated.

As you learn to breathe correctly you will notice that the hand upon your chest is still, with no rise and fall. You will notice, however, that the hand resting upon the abdomen will rise and fall as you find your own natural rhythm.

Continue to be aware of the rise and fall of your abdomen. Now focus on your breathing. Every time you breathe out think of the word . . . relax.

Inhale . . . *calm* . . . . Exhale . . . relax . . . you may prefer to breathe in and out through your nostrils once you have found your natural rhythm.

I will leave you for a few moments to enjoy the feeling of relaxation.

[Practise this exercise at least once a day; once mastered you will be able to enter into guided imagery, visualization and self-hypnosis.]

At peace with pain

[Allow time for diaphragmatic breathing before reading the script.]

Concentrate on your left arm . . . maybe you feel it getting heavy, so heavy but warm and comfortable, maybe you would like to lift your left arm, but it is so heavy and comfortable you may prefer not to. Your whole body feels heavy, warm and heavy, now concentrate on your right arm, so light . . . so light and fluffy, so light you may feel your right arm floating . . . gently up . . . so light and comfortable . . . maybe your right arm is so light you can gently raise it . . . maybe you would like to raise your right arm, maybe now your right arm has the same sensation as the rest of your body, warm . . . so warm . . . so heavy . . . so comfortable.

Your right arm, so heavy, you try to lift it but you cannot, because it is heavy and so comfortable . . . try to lift your right arm, say to yourself . . . my right arm is so heavy, so comfortable I may choose not to raise it.

The chair or floor is supporting your warm comfortable body and now knowing that you can move your right arm if you so wish you relax even deeper . . . pause.

Now we will take a journey . . . put behind you the self-hypnosis, concentrate on your breathing . . . . Inhale . . . . Relax.

Exhale . . . calm, inhale . . . relax, exhale . . . calm.

You begin your journey inward to the place where there is peace with pain.

You are in the midst of the swirling, screeching, wind and water, of the storm of pain . . . a giant hurricane that blows all around you.

You will pass through the storm to a place that is like the eye of a hurricane . . . where there is comfort and calm within the storm. You will travel across unfamiliar and challenging terrain to a special place.

You will move towards this place without map or compass, at times keenly aware of your surroundings . . . . At other times, just fixed on your goal . . . that special place within . . . where there is peace with pain.

You are driven with the power within you, which is greater than the fury of the storm of pain that swirls around you . . . seeking that special place within.

You begin your journey and travel on and on . . . on and on . . . on and on.

Now maybe you can focus on your journey, you travel on . . . until finally you arrive at the threshold of this place within.

A wooden door stands before you . . . . It has a deep rich grain that is so smooth.

You 'will' the door to open, focus on the door and 'will' it to open.

Your right hand is so light, maybe you open the door, yes the door opens.

You are transported away from the swirling, nagging, screeching, burning throbbing wall, to a calm quiet peaceful place.

You remain aware of the storm, but it seems far away.

Deep within you, you know that the harder the storm crashes . . . the harder it tears and flashes . . . the safer you become in this special place.

You are aware of your breathing . . . steady, calm, relaxed.

You are feeling calm and quiet.

As if in a deep sleep-like state, you feel secure and peaceful, aware and focused.

Now, aware of your surroundings, you notice that this place is strangely familiar . . . . At once it is both like a place you have been before and a place that is new to you . . . a place where you feel peace and calm . . . and where there are opportunities for you to discover the meaning of serenity.

Feeling calm and protected, you rest as if in a deep sleep-like state . . . like a deep, deep sleep, yet with a feeling of mental alertness. You feel secure and peaceful, aware and focused.

Moving further into this journey within . . . you hear the sound of the wind and water rise and fall . . . then fade away. The storm is swirling and crashing . . . pounding and flashing. Sometimes it seems near and sometimes it seems far away.

But here, in this place, you feel safe and secure . . . calm and peaceful . . . distant and detached from the fury of the storm that swirls around you.

You are unafraid and unhurt . . . and breathing in a way that is calm and relaxing . . . feeling a sense of serenity . . . feeling a special sense of inner peace.

You awaken as if within a dream to a new discovery . . . to the soothing power of warmth.

First you feel the warmth around you . . . very deep, very complete . . . feeling the warmth deep within you, feeling its soothing power.

Then maybe you notice that the storm has quieted. Less swirling . . . less and less fury . . . more gentle, more calm.

The warmth turns the raindrops to steam, and they evaporate before they touch the ground. The sun comes out . . . and shines its light through the rising steam.

You feel warm and soothed by the gentle mist.

Take some time now to feel that special feeling . . . calm . . . comfortable and relaxed
[Allow 10/12 seconds.]

Now you become aware of another soothing feeling . . . cooling . . . cool and refreshing . . . deep and almost numbing. You are now barely aware of the storm.

Sensing the cool and quiet . . . a faint swirling . . . now soft and gentle . . . you sense the 'cool' transforming the water of the storm . . . turning it to snow.

Bright sparkling snow crystals float in the air and reflect the light . . . then fall softly to the ground. A blanket of quiet white creates . . . a deep, deep restful sense of calm.

The whole landscape covered with snow . . . soft, smooth . . . makes you feel comfortable and relaxed . . . calm and at peace . . . no burning sensation, no intense pain . . . cool.

And peaceful . . . .
[Allow 10 seconds.]

In a moment you will prepare to leave your special place . . . but even as you think that thought, you feel secure in the knowledge that you can return at any time. Allow yourself to take something with you, something that will remind you of reaching inner peace and calm . . . something that will give you a sense of being special. Maybe it is the warm sun, melting the intensity of pain . . . maybe it is the cooling snow lessening the burning sensation . . . maybe it is the image of serenity, or peace of total relaxation.

This is your special place, it belongs only to you.

The more you journey to your special place . . . the easier it will be for you to find the way and the more comfortable and secure you will become . . . comfortable in the knowledge that you are able to sense a feeling of inner peace . . . pause . . . .

In a moment I will ask you to take a deep breath and to bring yourself back into this room. I will count from 1 to 3.
[Pause . . . with *a firm tone* . . .]

Now . . . take a deep breath . . . and blow it out.

1 . . . come back to the room.
2 . . . you feel calm and relaxed.
3 . . . as you open your eyes; you will feel rested and comfortable.

[This script incorporates autogenic statements. Adapted from John Heil, cited in Lusk (1993).]

Passive muscle relaxation (swimming in the sea)

You may want to start focusing on your breathing. When you take a breath in, your lungs start filling up with air. Allow the air to go all the way down to your stomach and as you are breathing out pretend that those feelings of tension that you may have begin to disappear. You may want to allow the relaxation to happen without forcing it. Don't worry about how well you are doing, allow the relaxation to flow over you, allow it to deepen at its own pace. Keep your breathing regular. Breathe in and out through your nose. Keep it steady and allow your breathing to find its own natural rhythm, very, very quiet and very still. Remember that the chair or the floor will give you all the support that your body needs so don't hold onto yourself. Remember that relaxation will make you healthier; it will give your brain time-out from tension and worry. It will release tension from your muscles, making you more efficient and productive; it will reduce your pain. Relax between your eyebrows and feel your forehead smoothing itself away. You may have your eyes closed and you might want to feel them sinking back into your head, quiet and still.

Pretend to focus on your breathing; when you take a breath in, your lungs start filling up with air. As you are breathing out, pretend that those feelings of tension that you may have leave your body. Breathe in and out and every time you do so pretend to relax a little more.

Now pretend that you take your mind to your right side, to your right leg and feel your right leg becoming heavier and heavier. Pretend that it is your right leg; if it is the left leg that you may want to concentrate on, that's OK. Sometimes when you relax you might not feel the difference between right and left. It feels so heavy that it starts to sink down into the chair/onto the floor. Your right leg, so heavy. So relax, gently sinking down into the chair. Now pretend that you are relaxing the other leg. It does not matter if it is the left or the right leg. It is becoming heavier and heavier. Your other leg is so heavy, so relaxed that it also begins to sink down into the chair. Both legs feel heavy, so heavy that you can hardly move them.

Now your hips; pretend that your hips feel heavy and they are so heavy and relaxed that they begin to sag into the chair/onto the floor.

You may want to concentrate on your arms. Feel your right arm. Whichever arm you choose to relax will start to feel heavy, heavier and more relaxed. You may want to move your fingers, to feel their touch against your legs or even the chair/the floor you are sinking into.

I invite you to do the same with the other arm; allow it to feel heavy, gently sinking into the chair. As you keep breathing in and out you are getting into a deeper level of relaxation. You may be hearing other people talking or even my voice. You are relaxing so well that it may not bother you whether I carry on or not helping you with relaxation.

Now pretend that you become aware of your shoulders and your back, pretend that they are heavy and feel them sinking, gently sinking. Now your whole body, your whole body, is so heavy, so relaxed. Allow yourself to go completely; your whole self sinking into the chair/onto the floor.

Now feel your inner self, floating upwards, your inner self gently floating upwards, floating upwards on a soft white cloud and drifting higher and higher, higher and higher up into the blue sky. Far below you, the countryside spreads out as far as you can see, as you drift lazily along on the soft white cloud.

As you float along, as you look below you, you may want to see a stream flowing down from the hills. You may see it, feel it or hear it and the white cloud begins to follow the stream. Pretend that other streams are joining you and becoming a small river. As it flows along, it goes through villages and as you look far below you, you see the houses and the people and the stream flows on becoming bigger and bigger. It goes through towns. You might want to see many houses and many people far, far below you. As you drift lazily along on your soft white cloud. Then in the distance you might pretend to see the coastline approaching and your river flows towards the coastline and gradually as you move close into the coastline, the river flows out into the ocean and you flow onwards far above the ocean on your soft white cloud, feeling the warmth of the sun above you.

And now you may want to travel to your special place, that place that is so special just for you. And now pretend that you are inside a glass tunnel. You may want to feel the touch of the glass with your fingers. Inside the tunnel you can hear the soothing music playing and you can pretend to see all the sea life swimming gracefully around you. Pretend to absorb the sheer serenity of this feeling of relaxation.

And now you may want to immerse yourself in the clear blue sea. Above you, you may imagine the sunny bright sky. Pretend that you can hear the sound of the waves and, as you feel the warm water around you, allow yourself to go to deeper levels of relaxation. And now allow yourself to feel the gentle movement, the water slowly and gently moving around you. Feel the gentle swimming of the dolphins and the smaller fish and the slow movement of the turtles. Allow the peaceful sound of the water to help you feel more deeply and deeply relaxed. Allow yourself to feel and touch the smooth skin of the dolphins. Pretend that your mind's eye can see the smaller more colourful fish swimming. It feels like the most beautiful display of different colours and, as you are looking up underneath the warm water, the sunshine on the surface is creating bright rainbows; the water is diffusing the light, creating bright rainbows. And now tell every nerve, every cell and every fibre in your body to release, relax and let go.

Allow the serenity, the peace and the joy to flow all over you and help you relax more and more.

I would like you to pretend that you enjoy the peace and serenity of your surroundings. Feel the positive energy of the sun above you and feel your whole self being renewed, revitalized and refreshed, your whole self being renewed, revitalized and refreshed. See yourself, as you would like to be. Pretend to feel that you are in perfect health, full of energy and any part of yourself that has not been functioning 100% efficiently, feel it as restored to normal functioning. See yourself as you would like to be. Enjoy this for a few minutes. Allow this thought to run through your mind, allow this thought to run through your mind.

I am going to start counting backwards from 5 to 1 and by the time I get to 1, you will feel relaxed and alert but fully refreshed. 5, 4, you may want to start moving your toes, 3, your fingers, 2 and 1. You may open your eyes.

[Adapted from an original script by psychologists Owen Hughes and Cristina López-Chertudi.]

CHAPTER EIGHT

Reactivation

JAN COOIL

Aim

To provide an overview of physical reactivation and how exercise links with and supports other pain-management strategies such as pacing and goal setting

Objectives

By the end of the chapter the reader will:

- be aware of patient and professional beliefs relating to exercise and chronic pain and the consequences of misconceptions and inaccurate messages;
- have an understanding of the physiological consequences of deconditioning and the positive effects of reconditioning;
- have an understanding of how to implement different types of exercise effectively;
- be aware of the issues that affect the selection of exercise including motivation and behavioural change, goal setting, specificity, quotas and pacing.

Introduction

Exercise is one of the most powerful weapons in the fight against chronic pain. Although it is a strong ally it is usually condemned as an enemy, something to be feared and avoided. This misconception, initiated through experiential learning by the patient, is often reinforced and perpetuated by the health professional. The result is the development of a vicious cycle of activity avoidance, declining fitness levels and activity intolerance, which

186

serves to reinforce the belief that exercise is harmful. The resultant reduction in physical ability may be accompanied by loss of social interaction, leading to a significant impact on the emotional state of the patient.

With a basic understanding of the relationship between exercise and chronic pain the health professional is in a position to empower the patient with some simple messages and straightforward strategies.

Patient misconceptions

Generally when people become ill or injured they assume an acute pain model. This is the most commonly understood model of pain in which the symptom is seen as a warning sign signifying tissue damage. The modifications made by patients following this model are entirely appropriate in the acute situation as they allow protection of the damaged tissue and healing to occur.

However, the expectation of becoming pain free is not always realistic. This is a difficult concept for the patient with chronic pain who believes that modern medicine will be able to 'fix the problem' and cure the pain. Where this fails to happen the patient usually believes that chronic pain is a sign of ongoing tissue damage.

Patients with chronic pain may respond in one of two ways: 'confrontation' or 'avoidance'. Confrontation is seen as an adaptive response to benign chronic pain and may result in the reduction of fear and pain and an increase in functional activity. Avoidance, on the other hand, is seen as a maladaptive response to benign chronic pain, which may result in amplification of fear and pain and a reduction in functional activity.

There appears to be a curvilinear association between anxiety and pain behaviour. Moderate levels of fear and anxiety have been shown as helpful by initiating coping strategies such as seeking information and advice; however, extreme levels of anxiety result in incapacitation. Moderate levels of fear and anxiety encourage thoughtful and effective action whereas high levels result in disordered and ineffective action.

A significant number of patients will adjust exceptionally well to a chronic pain state, requiring little in the way of healthcare (Linton, 1998). In comparison, though, a small number of people adjust badly and require a substantial amount of healthcare. Models have been proposed to explain why people develop chronic pain. The term 'kinesiophobia' was presented to describe 'an excessive, irrational and debilitating fear of physical movement and activity resulting from a feeling of vulnerability to painful injury or re-injury' (Kori et al., 1990). Lethem et al. (1983) described the 'fear-avoidance model of exaggerated pain perception' and Vlaeyen et al. (1995) developed a 'cognitive model of fear of movement and (re) injury'. All of these models described fear of pain or more specifically fear of pain that will result in (re)injury.

The fear avoidance exhibited by patients with chronic pain is said to be comparable to the behaviour seen in phobias. Learning appears to play a key part in how the patient adapts. Information gathered from a range of sources will develop beliefs, which in turn affect the emotions experienced by the individual. Patients who believe that their ongoing pain is a sign of progressive damage will learn to fear and avoid the pain. As physical activity often appears to exacerbate the pain, patients learn to avoid movements and activities. In the short term their behaviour may appear helpful in controlling and reducing the pain but in the long term avoidance is a maladaptive strategy, which serves to increase disability. Unfortunately short-term reinforcers tend to maintain the avoidance pattern. Resting and taking medication may serve to reduce pain and fear; pain behaviour is rewarded with attention and avoidance of unpleasant duties whereas passive activities such as watching the television may increase pleasure.

The shift in lifestyle is often so slow and subtle that the patient fails to see the changes taking place. Alongside the changes in function, emotional changes may occur. Patients may become depressed and passive as they begin to believe that there is little they can do to control the pain. Guilt may accompany a change in role within the family, low self-esteem may result from a change in body shape and anger and resentment are common responses to loss of ability. Thus a vicious cycle occurs in which the unhelpful beliefs lead to fear, fear leads to avoidance and avoidance results in reduced physical capacity. The reduction in physical capacity may increase depression and, as a result, lower the pain threshold and tolerance.

As avoidance tendencies within patients with chronic pain are associated with poor treatment outcomes it is important that health professionals give clear, accurate messages that reassure the patient and encourage the maintenance of function, including work.

See Chapter 5 for further discussion of this issue.

Professional beliefs and influences

There has been a significant amount of research examining avoidance behaviour in chronic pain patients, which attempts to identify the factors that cause the fear (Nicholas et al., 1992; Waddell et al., 1993). From these studies the health professional has been identified as a source of fear to such an extent that Waddell (1993) has described a large amount of chronic low back pain as being 'iatrogenic' or resulting from treatment.

Inaccurate information and inappropriate advice have been suggested as iatrogenic causes of chronicity in patients with chronic low back pain

(Harding and Williams, 1995; Rose, 1998). Taylor and Rose (1996) found that this notion was confirmed in the reports given by patients with chronic low back pain attending rehabilitation units. The preponderance of the patients in the study believed that their spine was diseased and at risk of injury.

Bedrest, activity restriction and analgesia comprise the past common medical management of low back pain. This approach is now widely condemned as it is both unhelpful and potentially harmful, suggesting to the patient that there are vulnerable tissues that require protection. Thus it appears that the clinician's beliefs are important as they influence the beliefs of the patient. Diagnosis, prognosis, descriptive language and behavioural advice are four of the main areas in which the health professional can communicate in an unhelpful way and some examples are highlighted below.

Biomedical diagnosis

If the health professional uses a medical model to explain pain there is the requirement to confirm a diagnosis – that is, find a tissue to blame. The major consequence of explaining a medical diagnosis to a patient appears to be that it creates misunderstanding and encourages fear-avoidance behaviour (Waddell et al., 1993).

A recent study explored the information patients were given regarding their chronic pain condition and their interpretation of this (Hafner, 2002). One of the main findings of this work was that health professionals often directly attribute the patient's pain to the degenerative changes identified on X-rays and scans. The accuracy of these professional beliefs remains unsubstantiated, however; patients often take this information to mean that they have a disease that is likely to be progressive. This belief inevitably leads to fear and avoidance behaviour.

Prognosis

Although some patients may assume a prognosis, many are given explicit indications of what the future is likely to hold by a health professional. An example of a prognosis that is occasionally given to young patients with significant spinal problems is: 'You will be in a wheelchair by the time you're forty.'

More often than not a patient will believe such a statement without question and change their behaviour in light of this 'fact'. Some will reduce and avoid activity in order to preserve their function in the future. Others may become overactive believing that they may not have the opportunity in the future. Some patients make major life choices, such as whether or when to have children, based on the prognosis they are given. Often patients are given information regarding the activities they will not be able to do in the future, such as lift weights. Such statements prove extremely influential despite the fact that there is little evidence to support their accuracy.

Imagery

The words that health professionals use to describe a disease or injury inevitably create a picture in the mind of the patient. Our words therefore have the power to invoke destructive as well as helpful images. Often simple language such as 'a slipped disc' will conjure up an image of the disc as a 'flying saucer' that has 'shot out of place' or 'crumbling spine' produces a picture of bones crumbling like a packet of biscuits. Words such as 'degenerative' may be taken to mean progressive joint failure and the soft tissues in injuries such as whiplash may be described as 'torn'. Thus, although unintentional, our own language could be described as catastrophic as it is interpreted as such by our patients.

Behavioural advice

Patients frequently misunderstand their pain and its relationship to disease or injury and healing. Such misunderstanding leads the patient to fear their pain and its implication. Unfortunately health professionals often inadvertently reinforce this fear in the behavioural advice that they offer. The most common reinforcer is the advice to rest. The use of rest and its relationship to tissue damage and pain are poorly explained, if at all. Patients will assume that if they need to rest then there must be something significantly wrong. Patients who are told to rest may not be told how they should limit the rest and progress activity. Where patients are given instruction they are often told to 'let pain be your guide'.

Even in acute conditions pain is only partly related to tissue damage and thus fails as a useful symptom by which to guide reactivation. The instruction to let pain be your guide will reinforce avoidance of activities that are painful thereby encouraging fear-avoidance behaviour. Therapists involved in rehabilitating a patient may also fear exacerbating the patient's pain. Where there is an increase in pain in relation to an activity or exercise, such a fear will influence the therapist to reduce, stop or change their rehabilitation plan. Again this gives a clear message to the patient that the increase in pain signifies that something is wrong and that this should be avoided.

A common belief among health professionals is that primarily patients wish to receive information relating to the diagnosis and cause of their pain. Von Korff and Saunders (1996) undertook a study of patients with a first episode of back pain and found that the participants identified several other matters as more important. The participants wished to know the expected course of their back pain and how to deal with the problem, their activity restrictions, how to return to normal as quickly as possible and, finally, how to reduce the likelihood and intensity of future episodes.

Despite the fact that these findings indicate that patients want to learn how to manage their pain, health professionals often fail to provide the information necessary for this. One of the most common examples within chronic pain is the advice, 'learn to live with it'. In the words of P. Moore, an ex-INPUT graduate and expert patient programme tutor: 'They say learn to live with it but don't tell you how. That's like saying go home and bake a cake but without giving you the recipe or the ingredients.'

It doesn't take a lot of imagination to understand how frustrating and disempowering this must be. Indeed, if patients wish for this information then surely they must be 'active copers' when they do so, but without the relevant advice they may be relegated by health professionals to the role of the 'passive patients'.

As an alternative the health professional should ensure that their own beliefs are accurate and are communicated in a helpful and understandable manner to the patient, taking into consideration that patients' beliefs and comprehension contribute to their successful management (Linton, 1998) by allowing demedicalization of the condition and basic changes to be made to the patient's beliefs.

Deconditioning

Physical activity is essential for the maintenance of physical function. When the body is denied activity, through illness or injury, two major physical effects are seen. The first is a loss of fitness specific to the compromised body part due to internal (for example, muscular) or external (for example, a cast or brace) protection or immobilization. The second effect is a more widespread loss of fitness as a consequence of a general reduction in activity.

As previously discussed, some patients with chronic pain avoid activity and exercise and this results in the secondary impairment of deconditioning. Astrand and Rodahl (1986) defined deconditioning as 'a loss of aerobic capacity or physical work capacity'. As fitness levels reduce so does tolerance of exercise and therefore patients will experience pain at increasingly lower activity levels. Reduced activity tolerance leads to greater anxiety and fear avoidance, and thus a vicious cycle develops. Deconditioning and activity intolerance are a principal cause of disability in the patient with chronic pain and may lead to new pains from weakness, tightness, abnormal movement patterns and increased states of tension.

Musculoskeletal changes

A reduction in activity levels causes a reduction in the strength and mass of all tissues in the musculoskeletal system (Twomey, 1992).

Bone

Bone requires repeated stress, particularly weight-bearing stress, to encourage remodelling and increased density. In the absence of such stress there is no demand for strength and bone density decreases.

Muscle

Muscle will begin to lose both flexibility and strength as quickly as 24 hours following immobilization. Without normal movement muscle will fail to be stretched and as a result will adaptively shorten, leading to a loss of range of motion. Muscles that are particularly prone to contracture are those that cross more than one joint such as the hamstrings. These changes are usually reversible with an appropriate programme of stretching exercises.

Muscle strength may be reduced by three mechanisms:

1. A muscle that has shortened is no longer able to produce peak tension and develops 'tight weakness'.
2. With a reduced demand for contraction, muscle fibres atrophy, leading to a loss of strength. This is particularly so in the slow twitch fibres, which over time reduce in number and develop fast twitch characteristics.
3. Motor neuron discharge is decreased as a result of immobilization.

Connective tissue

Connective tissue such as tendons, ligaments, fascia and joint capsules requires frequent motion to boost its metabolism and remodelling. Collagen is the structure that absorbs the majority of stress within connective tissue, whilst elastin provides compliance. The greater the proportion of collagen fibres, arranged in parallel fashion, the greater the tensile strength of the tissue.

With reduction of stress, due to inactivity, there is a reduction in the size and number of collagen fibres resulting in connective tissue weakness. In addition the proportion of elastin fibres increases resulting in greater compliance. Further, where a tissue is immobilized additional changes include weakening of the collagen, a decline in parallel orientation, a reduction in lubrication and an increase in adhesions. Adhesions, which will reduce range of motion, may also occur as the result of scar tissue formation following injury or fibrotic changes as a result of chronic inflammation. The effects of inactivity and immobilization on connective tissue may be avoided or lessened with appropriate exercise. Recovery of tensile strength may take as long as 12 months.

Intervertebral disc

Spinal movement ensures that fluid exchange occurs between the intervertebral discs and the surrounding interstitial fluid. Thus, the intervertebral disc, like the other tissues, also relies on movement to maintain nutrition.

Articular cartilage

Movement ensures that synovial fluid passes over the articular cartilage of the joint and alternate compression loading and unloading of a joint encourage it to pass into the articular cartilage (Twomey, 1992). This process is essential for the nutrition of the articular cartilage. Immobility may therefore result in a lack of nutrition and subsequent cartilage degeneration.

Cardiovascular and respiratory changes

Immobilization also produces unfavourable effects within the cardiovascular system. For every day of immobilization the resting heart rate increases by a half beat per minute. Alongside this increase in heart rate, the stroke rate, distal volume, vital capacity and maximum oxygen uptake all reduce.

The cardiovascular system of inactive individuals responds in a similar way with an increase in resting heart rate and a poor oxygen delivery system. The muscular changes described above also affect the respiratory muscles resulting in an inability to take deeper and more frequent breaths. Low levels of aerobic exercise provoke a disproportionate cardiovascular response in unfit individuals so that they quickly experience shortness of breath and fatigue and find it tough to maintain a constant workload without exhaustion. As there is reduced oxygen availability, the working muscles switch their energy supply to carbohydrates resulting in the production of lactic acid. The build-up of lactate reduces the ability of the muscle to contract and quickly leads to fatigue and pain.

Neurophysiological changes

Proprioception is the ability to know body position. The information required for this skill is provided by sensory receptors within the muscles, ligaments and joint capsules. The proprioceptors within the capsule and ligaments are stimulated by force or strain applied to the joint. The muscles that control the joint will then work together to provide dynamic stabilization. The proprioceptive systems may be impaired either through direct injury or by long-standing disuse. Thus lack of proprioceptive sense will limit normal reflex stabilization of joints, giving rise to a reduction in balance and skill and a greater potential for injury and degeneration (Barrett et al., 1991).

Reconditioning

An appropriate programme of exercise can avoid or reverse most of the effects of immobilization or inactivity. According to Wolff's law, in which a change in form follows a change in function, bones react to normal activities or increased stress by preserving or developing their strength. This is due to the electrical potential that is developed at sites of compression and tension influencing osteoclastic and osteoblastic activity to increase bone density. Connective tissue responds in a similar fashion to bone, with increased stress resulting in greater density and consequently greater tissue strength.

Muscles that are stretched regularly will respond by maintaining or increasing their length and those that are subject to regular resistive loading develop greater cross-sectional width, blood and nerve supply and hence increased strength. Gentle repetitive movement of the peripheral and spinal joints will result in greater nutrition of the articular cartilage and intervertebral discs.

Cardiovascular fitness may be improved by working the body's large muscle groups over an adequate period of time on a regular basis. For the deconditioned individual, as this requires working aerobically, exercises would be performed at a low level. Regular aerobic activity will result in a lower resting heart rate and improvement in aerobic capacity.

Exercise planning

Different types of exercise, therefore, will address the different deficits created by fear avoidance and the subsequent deconditioning of the patient with chronic pain. It is useful to link a programme of exercise and activity to the patient's specific needs and functional deficits via a process of goal and quota setting. For ease of description exercise has been broadly divided into:

- flexibility;
- strength;
- aerobic work.

It is important to recognize, however, that most functional activities require a combination of these abilities. Prior to undertaking any exercise it is helpful to warm up, and following the exercise cool down.

Flexibility

Flexibility is defined as the range of movement at a specific joint or group of joints. The related bones, soft tissue structures such as muscles, tendons and ligaments and other collagenous structures around the joint, such as fascia, control flexibility. Good flexibility demonstrates a lack of contractures or adhesions in the supporting soft tissues.

As previously highlighted soft tissue shortening may arise as a result of tissue injury, immobilization or restricted mobility, activity avoidance and poor posture. As a consequence the individual will develop stiff joints and tight muscles resulting in a loss of flexibility.

Complete, unlimited movement is an important element of physical fitness. An effective flexibility programme should aim to increase the range of movement, particularly of affected joints, by improving the elasticity of the soft tissue structures that pass across the joint. Stretching is described as a rehabilitative movement intended to lengthen contracted soft tissue structures and thus increase range of movement.

Therapeutic effects of flexibility

It is well established that soft tissues that are consistently stretched over a considerable length of time adapt by lengthening. This allows a greater range of movement to occur at the joints affected by those tissues. Such an increase in flexibility has been shown to lead to improved physical performance. With greater flexibility an individual is able to move without restriction thereby allowing freer and easier movement. This allows the body to use the most efficient and effective movement patterns employing greater strength, balance and coordination. Stretching exercises may make strenuous activities easier as they prepare the body for activity.

The risk of injury may be reduced with greater flexibility. If the soft tissues have good elasticity they are less easily overstretched or torn, the individual is able to change direction more easily and is less likely to be injured should they fall. Stretching exercises may also lower muscle tension giving an enhanced state of relaxation.

Types of stretch

Contractile tissue (muscle) and non-contractile tissue (ligaments, fascia and so forth) are the two types of soft tissue structures that control joint motion. These tissues have distinctive properties that affect their ability to lengthen. Contractile and non-contractile tissues both have elastic and plastic properties. The ability of a soft tissue to return to its resting length following the application of a stretch force is termed elasticity. The ability of a soft tissue to lengthen following the application of a stretch force is termed plasticity. Stretching techniques have developed over time. Three main approaches to stretching have emerged:

1. Ballistic stretching is the oldest approach to stretching. It involves making small-amplitude, high-velocity movements – short, bouncing movements – at the end of available joint range or muscle length.
2. Static stretching involves moving to the end of available joint range or muscle length and maintaining that position, without moving, for a longer period of time.
3. Proprioceptive neuromuscular facilitation (PNF) comprises a group of techniques which involves alternate phases of muscle contraction and relaxation at the end of available joint range or muscle length. Contract-relax, hold-relax and slow reversals are the most commonly used techniques.

All of these involve a 5- to 10-second contraction against resistance at the end of range followed by a similar period of relaxation. All three stretching techniques have been shown to increase soft muscle length. There is debate, however, as to which technique is the most effective at improving flexibility.

How to stretch

It is important to inform the patient that bouncing up and down is the wrong way to stretch as this can actually do more harm than good. A slow, sustained stretch is safe and effective as it is less likely to initiate the stretch reflex and increase muscle tension. In addition this stretch should be gentle, performed at a position of comfortable tension rather than pain. It may be useful to inform the patient that it is better to under-stretch than to over-stretch as relaxation and consistency are more important features of a successful stretching programme.

Stretching techniques are performed more safely and effectively if the soft tissues involved are warm. Therefore it is wise to undertake some gentle active exercise prior to stretching in order to increase the body temperature. Alternatively superficial heat could be applied to the soft tissues involved. For a more thorough explanation of superficial heating and soft tissue flexibility refer to Chapter 9.

As it is important to be as relaxed as possible, breathing should be slow, controlled and fluid with each of the stretch positions described. When moving into the position of stretch the patient should breathe out and then, in the stretch, breathe slowly while the position is maintained. If the position of the stretch inhibits breathing then it must be recognized that the patient will not be relaxed. If breathing is inhibited it is helpful to reduce the stretch to allow a relaxed breathing pattern to occur.

The first stretch should be an easy stretch where the patient moves to and then maintains a position of mild muscle tension but is able to remain relaxed. Following the easy stretch the patient may then repeat the manoeuvre but move to and maintain a position of moderate stretch. The patient should feel greater muscle tension in this position but should still remain comfortable. This is often called a developmental stretch (Anderson, 1981).

There is no one ideal time of the day at which to stretch. It is more important to identify a time of the day that is appropriate to the patient. Often patients feel stiff first thing in the morning in which case stretching could be employed following a hot bath or shower to ease out stiff joints and muscles. There are many activities during the day that may lead to a feeling of stiffness, for example sitting or standing for a long time or doing a repetitive activity such as typing. In these cases stretching may help to ease tension in the affected muscles. Similarly, stretching may be useful to relieve muscle tension at times of anxiety. Stretching helps prepare the body for more strenuous physical activity and is also useful as part of a cool down to avoid stiffness.

There are two 'traps' that patients often fall into – they compare themselves with themselves and with others. To address these it is useful to let the patient know that they should expect to be different every day and whether they feel tight and stiff or loose and relaxed they should still stretch following the principles outlined above. In addition, as each person has differing natural and acquired levels of flexibility, it is unhelpful and potentially misleading to use a comparison with others.

Strength

Strength is defined as 'the ability of the musculoskeletal system to produce force' (Asanovich, 1992). Power is the ability of the body to generate a high force over a short time. Endurance is the ability of the body to generate a low force over a long time. Thus strength training is the process of improving or increasing the body's ability to generate force and uses movements that are performed against resistance.

Although strength is an essential component of physical fitness, it may be lost incredibly quickly as a result of immobilization or inactivity. A loss of muscle strength has a significant impact on functional capacity. Therefore strength training may be an important consideration in the functional rehabilitation of the patient with chronic pain.

Therapeutic effects of strength

Muscles that are worked against resistance on a regular basis over sufficient time will respond by becoming stronger. Greater strength will improve both power and endurance and will increase the functional ability of the body to, for example, push, pull and lift. Improved muscle strength allows for a more efficient posture and a greater level of joint protection, which may prove of huge benefit to the patient with chronic pain.

Muscle tissue burns energy even when at rest. Thus the more a body is composed of muscle the more energy it requires and the higher its metabolic rate. This is an important factor in weight control as strengthening exercises may be used as a complementary strategy to cardiovascular work for those patients who wish to control weight or as an alternative strategy for those patients who find cardiovascular work difficult.

Types of muscle contraction

There are several types of muscle contraction that may be used within muscle-strengthening exercises:

- An isometric contraction occurs when a muscle contracts in a static position, that is, the length of the muscle and the angle of the joint remain unchanged. An isometric contraction would occur where a muscle works statically against an object that cannot be moved.
- An isotonic contraction occurs when a muscle contracts producing movement of the body part through the available joint range while maintaining a constant tension. Exercise that produces such contraction has the value of working the muscles through their full range without the need for expensive equipment.

- An isokinetic contraction occurs when a muscle contracts producing movement of the body part through available joint range while maintaining a constant velocity. Exercise that produces such contraction requires the use of isokinetic machines, which are not usually available in leisure centres and are therefore not practical for most people.

Both isotonic and isokinetic exercises may occur as concentric or eccentric contractions:

- A concentric contraction occurs when a muscle shortens against a load.
- An eccentric contraction occurs when a muscle lengthens against a load.

For example, if a weight is held in the hand with the arm by the side of the body, a concentric contraction of the biceps muscle will occur to bend the elbow and lift the weight. When the same weight is lowered by allowing the elbow to straighten, an eccentric contraction of the biceps muscle will occur.

Exercises that work the muscles through their full range are functionally valuable. There is, however, a place for isometric exercise, most notably when a body part is immobilized, for example in plaster, denying the individual the opportunity to work through the full range.

Resistance

Although weights are the type of resistance most often thought about when considering strength training, there are many more approaches to exercise that offer resistance. Elastic exercise bands have become popular and offer a cost-effective, portable and versatile means of strength training. Water provides both a supportive and a resistive medium for exercise. Callisthenics (free exercise) uses the resistance offered by body parts, lever lengths and gravity. The traditional press-up is a good example of a free exercise that uses the weight of the body against the effects of gravity for resistance. Lifting the uppermost leg when in the side-lying position uses the resistance offered by lifting a body part against gravity. If, in the previous exercise, the leg is bent, the lever length and therefore the load are reduced. In addition, if the position is changed to supine lying gravity becomes neutral to the muscle that brings the leg out to the side.

Types of strength

In order to develop greater strength it is essential to increase the workload placed upon a muscle or body part. This may be achieved by increasing the resistive load, the speed of the loaded movement, the number of loaded repetitions or a combination of these factors. Power is increased in muscles by moving a high resistance a few times. Endurance is increased in muscles by moving a low resistance a large number of times. Muscle strength and endurance are closely related. As strength improves there is a resultant increase in endurance as the load becomes easier to move. Therefore an improvement in strength is accompanied by a corresponding gain, not only in muscle power but also in speed and endurance. Moreover, a gain in muscular strength is associated with an increase in the capacity of the body to make quick, coordinated movements.

How to strengthen

As with stretching, it is important that the individual undertakes a warm-up prior to engaging in strengthening exercises. If isometric exercises are used then ideally a maximal contraction of 6 seconds should be repeated 5 to 10 times per session and sessions should be repeated daily. To be effective, isotonic exercises should be performed through the full range of joint motion, moving smoothly through the concentric phase of the exercise and returning more slowly through the eccentric phase. The most common approach is to perform sets of 10 exercises that are repeated two or three times. The strengthening session is then repeated daily or on alternate days.

When determining the number of repetitions and sets of strengthening exercises it is important to temper common practice with common sense in the beginning, and perform only a few exercises with a light resistance. This is a useful strategy to avoid delayed-onset muscle soreness, where pain and stiffness due to connective tissue inflammation and muscle swelling follow exercise as a result of working beyond muscle tolerance. Once a manageable starting point has been established it is a simple task to build up the resistance and number of repetitions in a slow and structured manner.

Aerobic fitness

Aerobic fitness may be described as an individual's ability to carry out prolonged types of physical activity. It is also called cardiorespiratory or cardiovascular fitness and includes the ability of the respiratory and circulatory systems to adapt to and recover from moderate-to-brisk activities.

Inactivity and rest result in a reduction in capacity within the respiratory and cardiovascular systems resulting in intolerance for low levels of aerobic workload. Aerobic exercise is designed to increase the respiratory, cardiac and circulatory systems' ability to take in, transport and use oxygen, thereby allowing the body to undertake energetic activities over extended periods of time.

Therapeutic effects of aerobic fitness

Regular aerobic exercise increases the efficiency of the respiratory muscles so that a greater lung capacity may be used during exercise. Endurance training reduces both the resting and the working heart rate and increases the stroke volume, and blood volume and total haemoglobin increase with training, swelling the capacity of the oxygen transport system.

Aerobic training has three main effects on muscle:

1. It increases the levels of enzymes required for the aerobic breakdown of fuel for energy;
2. It increases the size and number of mitochondria that produce energy aerobically;
3. It increases the muscle's ability to use fat as an energy source.

Not only is muscle contraction improved but fat mobilization is also increased. Undertaking a regular programme of aerobic exercise also results in improved efficiency and economy of motion in relation to the practised activity. Moderate activity causes an increase in bone density and the soft tissues respond to the stresses placed upon them by becoming stronger.

Evidence shows that, with increased exercise, anxiety and depression are reduced. People who exercise on a regular basis tend to fall asleep more quickly than inactive people, spend more time in slow-wave sleep and feel less tired in the morning.

Exercise parameters

To attain aerobic fitness it is important to raise the metabolic rate and the oxygen consumption of muscles and sustain this level for sufficient time to overload the aerobic enzyme systems (Sharkey, 1990). Workload, then, has to exceed a minimum level (training threshold) if adjustments in fitness are to take place. However, workload also has a maximum level (anaerobic threshold) beyond which training becomes primarily anaerobic. This is unhelpful as it does overload the aerobic systems. Therefore to improve aerobic fitness it is important to stay in the aerobic training zone.

In the inactive and unfit individual both the training and the anaerobic thresholds are lower than in the trained individual. Therefore unfit individuals can work and make progress at a lower intensity than their fitter peers. Both heart rate and perceived exertion have been used to quantify training intensity.

Studies appear to agree that workload intensity has to exceed a heart rate of 130 beats per minute. As unfit individuals will have a higher resting heart rate and will respond with more exaggerated increases than the fit individual, a lower level of activity would be required for them to reach this point.

Perceived exertion scales have been developed by Dr Gunnar Borg, a Swedish psychologist, and are currently used in many forms of exercise. Borg (1973) worked with the understanding that the brain, in the perception of effort, integrates sensory stimuli from the respiratory, cardiovascular and musculoskeletal systems. Subsequent studies have shown that subjective perception of effort correlates closely to workload, heart rate and oxygen consumption and is therefore a reasonable estimate of exercise intensity. A subjective rating of 'somewhat hard' is approximately equal to a heart rate of 130 beats per minute. It may be useful for patients, rather than focusing on their pain symptoms, to concentrate on their perception of warmth, heart rate and respiratory effort. Although aerobic exercise should feel somewhat hard, the individual should still be able to continue a conversation.

Duration is inversely related to intensity. An increase in one requires a decrease in the other. It is possible to measure duration in terms of time, distance or energy consumption. Patients with chronic pain, who have become unfit, will be able to work neither at high intensity nor for long duration. However it has been shown that low intensity exercise of 5–10 minutes is sufficient to improve fitness in the inactive individual (Sharkey, 1990). As fitness increases, duration may be increased to encourage greater fitness gains.

The frequency of sessions per week will, again, vary with the fitness of the individual. For the unfit, two to three sessions per week have been shown to improve fitness. However, as fitness improves, frequency must also increase if continued improvements are to be made and ideally the individual should aim for six sessions per week.

Warm-up

The process of warming up prior to undertaking an activity or exercise of moderate intensity remains the subject of ongoing study. As, in the main, evidence tends to support its use it is prudent to understand its potential value for the patient with chronic pain (Table 8.1).

Physiological changes during warm-up

With a rise in body temperature there are corresponding changes in circulation. Vasodilatation occurs in the areas that are used to undertake the activity – that is, the working muscles. Vasoconstriction occurs in the areas that are not required for the activity – for example, the gastrointestinal tract. As temperature increases within the soft tissues, the collagenous structures respond by becoming more elastic. The volume of synovial fluid

Table 8.1 Warm-up and cool-down technique

Warm-up	Cool-down
Time differs – increases with age 15–30 min	Follows main activity Should last 10 min
Increase activity sufficient to prepare the body for exercise	Gradual dwindling of work intensity

Progressive in nature:
  General exercise (marching on spot)
  Rhythmical
  Continuous
  Increasing in intensity
	As activity decreases:
	  Blood redistributes – reduces flow
	    to muscles, increases flow to
	    other areas
	  Reduces work of heart and muscle
	    pump
	  Gentle stretching reduces muscle
	    soreness

Increase tempo from moderate pace until body is warm, and heart and respiratory rate increased	Should follow format of the warm-up but in opposite way – reduce intensity to leisurely pace
May not be realistic for chronic pain at present fitness level – start slow and small and build up	

(joint lubricant) is increased and its viscosity is reduced resulting in improved joint lubrication. Both blood sugar and adrenaline (epinephrine) are mobilized in readiness for exercise.

Therapeutic effects of warming up

Warming up is believed to protect the soft tissues from strains and sprains. As the soft tissues become more elastic the potential for muscle tears and ligamentous strains is reduced. It is also believed that muscle soreness is prevented when the body is prepared for activity. In addition warming up the muscles specific to the activity to be undertaken results in an improvement in coordination and agility.

Exercise selection

Patients with chronic pain are nearly always unfit, with poor flexibility, reduced muscle strength and endurance and decreased aerobic capacity. A programme of physical activity is therefore important to include within daily activities in order to address specific impairments and lack of functional ability. Exercise selection may appear difficult as the patient often has a multitude of needs.

Motivation

Kerns et al. (1997) outlined a psychological tool that could be used to measure inclination to change within patients with chronic pain. They described four stages of patient readiness to adopt a self-management approach:

1. Pre-contemplation – it may be useful to discuss the relationship between pain and exercise, in particular that an increase in pain does not indicate an increase in damage, in order to effect a shift to the stage of contemplation.
2. Contemplation – patients may find it helpful to have clear advice on the benefits of exercise and how to achieve this so that they are able to shift towards action.
3. Action – patients may find advice on exercise progression or variation useful.
4. Maintenance – patients may find it useful to reassess and redefine their goals in order to keep their interest and ensure that they maintain their activity.

Rehabilitation success may therefore be improved by matching advice to the patient's motivational level.

Self-efficacy

Bandura (1977) defined self-efficacy as 'people's judgements of their capacities to organize and execute courses of action required to attain designated types of performances' and highlighted that confidence is not a general attribute but is specific to the situation we find ourselves in. Several studies, including one into exercise adherence, have shown that self-efficacy does predict behaviour. Therefore it is important to recognize that inactive pain patients may have little confidence in their ability to carry out a programme of exercise. Selecting an environment and activity that are non-threatening and provide the patient with positive, unconditional verbal encouragement may enhance success.

Attitude

Of all the attitudinal perspectives, the theory of planned behaviour (Fishbein and Ajzen, 1977) is possibly the most important in relation to exercise adherence. This highlights the importance of examining attitudes that relate to specific behavioural targets. That is, rather than looking at the attitude to exercise, it is more useful to look at the attitude to performing, for example, a hamstring-stretching programme every morning before getting out of bed. They argued that behaviour could then be predicted by examining the combination of behavioural intention, attitude, perceived behavioural control and social norms.

Thus, patients who are likely to adhere to the hamstring-stretching programme are those who state their intent to do so, believe it would benefit them, feel confident that they will be able to carry it out and identify that the people important to them wish for them to do so. In contrast, patients who are unlikely to adhere to the hamstring-stretching programme decline to undertake the programme, do not believe that it will be helpful, lack confidence that they will be able to succeed with it and identify that the people important to them either do not care or do not wish them to undertake the programme.

It is important to establish that patients wish to undertake the prescribed activity, feel confident to do so and believe that it will benefit them. In addition it is useful to ensure that the people important to them, which may include other health professionals, friends, family or colleagues, also believe the same.

Goals

The acronym SMARTER may be used for goal setting:

- specific;
- measurable;
- achievable;
- relevant;
- time limited;
- evaluated;
- rewarded.

Making goals specific, measurable and time limited may assess the patient's attitude to the planned behaviour. Discussing whether the goal is achievable may assess their confidence and perceived control. Those patients who are currently active and maintaining a programme of exercise may find ongoing motivation through the process of evaluation and reward. Relevance is pivotal to patient-centred care.

Often the health professional may use a therapist-centred approach, which involves detecting the patient's impairments and identifying a programme of exercises aimed at resolving these. This, however, runs the risk of disengaging the patient from the process. More likely to succeed is a patient-centred approach, in which patients select the impairment or function they would most like to improve and the health professional identifies a programme of activity to address this.

To facilitate this process it is useful to ask a patient to identify on a checklist why they wish to become more active (see Appendix on page 209). The answers may be surprising, with patients often wishing to feel better about themselves, socialize and reduce tension rather than become fitter or healthier. Completing such a checklist will enable the health professional to determine the most appropriate type of exercise or environment.

Specificity

The outcomes of an exercise programme correlate directly to the activities undertaken. This is known as specificity. It means that engaging in an activity such as walking recruits muscle fibres, metabolic pathways and energy sources appropriate to that task. By walking on a regular basis these fibres and pathways are recruited time after time and the body responds with an adaptive response known as the training effect. The training effect is specific to the task repeated; in other words, the training effects of a walking programme will not transfer to cycling or swimming. Although training effects are specific to the muscles recruited during the activity, some of the cardiovascular and respiratory effects will transfer and be generalized to other activities.

Given that training is specific, to improve a given functional activity it is important that the task itself is used as the basis for exercise. If a patient wishes to be able to kick a ball, for instance, then kicking a ball is the ideal exercise. If the activity is beyond the individual's current capabilities breaking it down into its individual components may phase it in. Each component may then be practised in turn, for example, standing on one leg, lifting the leg forward in standing and so on. Using a lighter ball and starting with only a few repetitions will also modify the duration and intensity of the task.

Quotas and pacing

Patients with chronic pain often appear to lack pacing skills. Any exercise-related experience generally falls within the 'no pain, no gain' type of underactivity/overactivity cycle. Although it is useful to inform the patient that it is normal to experience an increase in pain initially, pain is not used as a guide for quantifying exercise.

The tolerance of the patient for the agreed activity is assessed and a starting point is set well below tolerance. Exercise is then carried out regularly at this level. At preset times small increments are made to the base amount and exercise continues at this new and increased level. Patients should maintain a record of the resistance, repetitions or duration of their exercise.

This quota-based approach to exercise is important for two main reasons. First, if patients were to exercise to tolerance their symptoms, usually pain, will occur prior to the termination of exercise. This ensures that patients maintain their negative relationship between pain and exercise. Secondly, quota-based exercise allows the patient to initiate work and progress at a level that is within their individual capabilities and thus this approach divorces the pain from the activity.

Conclusion

This chapter has demonstrated the need for chronic pain patients to understand that if they 'don't use it, they will lose it'. As health professionals we have a duty of care to enable chronic pain patients to understand the importance of using their body to help control their pain: the correct use of language to prevent catastrophizing by the patient, the application of simple exercise regimes and identifying that to improve their pain they may after a small initial increase in pain begin to develop a sense of control and confidence, which will lead to a reduction in movement-related fear. Through this process patients will learn to take back control of some of the elements of their lives that had previously been lost to chronic pain.

References

Anderson B (1981) Stretching. London: Pelham Books.

Asanovich M (1992) What is strength? Athletic Conditioning Quarterly 1(1): 4–5.

Astrand P, Rodahl K (1986) Textbook of Work Physiology, Physiological Base of Exercise, 3rd edn. New York: McGraw-Hill.

Bandura A (1977) Self-efficacy: towards a unifying theory of behavioural change. Psychology Review 84: 191–215.

Barrett DS, Cobb AG, Bentley G (1991) Joint proprioception in normal, osteoarthritic and replaced knees. Journal of Bone and Joint Surgery 73B: 53–6.

Borg G (1973) Perceived exertion: a note on history and methods. Medicine and Science in Sports 5: 90–3.

Fishbein M, Ajzen I (1977) Attitude-behaviour relations: a theoretical analysis and review of the empirical research. Psychological Bulletin 84: 888–918.

Hafner C (2002) The information we give may be detrimental. In Gifford I (ed.) Topical Issues in Pain 4. Falmouth: CNS Press.

Harding V, Williams A de C (1995) Extending physiotherapy skills using a psychological approach: cognitive behavioural management of chronic pain. Physiotherapy 81: 681–8.

Kerns RD, Rosenberg R, Jamison RN et al. (1997) Readiness to adopt a self-management approach to chronic pain: the Pain Stages of Change Questionnaire (PSOCQ). Pain 72: 227–34.

Kori SH, Miller RP, Todd DD (1990) Kinesiophobia: a new view of chronic pain behaviour. Pain Management Jan/Feb: 35–43.

Lethem J, Slade PD, Troup JDG, Bentley G (1983) The fear avoidance model of exaggerated pain perception – 1. Behaviour Research and Therapy 21: 401–8.

Linton SJ (1998) The socioeconomic impact of chronic back pain: is anyone benefiting? Pain 75: 163–8.

Nicholas MK, Wilson PH, Goyen J (1992) Comparison of cognitive behavioural group treatment and an alternative non-psychological treatment for chronic low back pain. Pain 48: 339–47.

Rose M (1998) Iatrogenic disability and back pain rehabilitation. In Gifford L (ed.) Topical Issues in Pain 1. Falmouth: CNS Press.

Sharkey BJ (1990) Physiology of Fitness, 3rd edn. Champaign, IL: Human Kinetics Books.

Taylor D, Rose M (1996) Psychophysiological and psychological techniques for the treatment of low back pain. In Adams N (ed.) The Psychophysiology of Low Back Pain. New York: Churchill Livingstone.

Twomey LA (1992) A rationale for the treatment of back pain and joint pain by manual therapy. Physical Therapy 72: 885–92.

Vlaeyen JWS, Kole-Snijders AMJ, Boeren RGB, Van Eek H (1995) Fear of movement/(re) injury in chronic low back pain and its relationship to behavioural performance. Pain 62: 363–72.

Von Korff M, Saunders K (1996) The course of back pain in primary care. Spine 21: 2833–9.

Waddell, G, Newton, M, Henderson I et al. (1993) A fear-avoidance beliefs questionnaire (FABQ) and the role of fear-avoidance beliefs in chronic low back pain and disability. Pain 52: 157–68.

Appendix: Why do you want to become more active?

	Tick the statements that apply to you	**Which are the three most important ones?**
I want to . . .		
Improve my body shape	☐	☐
Gain or lose weight	☐	☐
Look and feel younger	☐	☐
Stay or get healthier	☐	☐
Keep or get fitter	☐	☐
Reduce my tension	☐	☐
Feel good about myself	☐	☐
Forget my worries	☐	☐
Increase my self awareness	☐	☐
Be challenged	☐	☐
Take my mind off work	☐	☐
Let off steam	☐	☐
Have time for myself	☐	☐
Make new friends	☐	☐
Spend time with others	☐	☐
Compete	☐	☐
Get away from people	☐	☐
Be part of a group	☐	☐

CHAPTER NINE

Self-treatment strategies

JAN COOIL

Aim

To provide an overview of the therapeutic effects of cutaneous stimulation strategies, their safe application and their relationship with other pain-management strategies.

Objectives

By the end of the chapter the reader will:

- understand the physiological and therapeutic effects of superficial heating and cooling and be aware of indications and contraindications for use and safe and simple methods of application;
- understand the physiological and therapeutic effects of massage and be aware of indications and contraindications for use and safe and simple methods of self-massage;
- understand the physiological and therapeutic effects of transcutaneous electrical nerve stimulation and be aware of indications and contraindications for use and safe and simple methods of application;
- be able to discuss appropriate treatment selection, highlighting the potential advantages of combination strategies.

Introduction

Heat, cold, massage and transcutaneous electrical nerve stimulation (TENS) have evolved from folk medicine into contemporary physical therapy modalities (Melzack, 1994: 1210). Although technology has developed sophisticated machines that heat, cool, move or stimulate body tissues, these advances have one common drawback for the chronic pain patient.

The more sophisticated the machine, the less it requires from the patient who is inevitably a passive recipient of such care and solely reliant on the treating clinician for this therapy.

Far more useful to the chronic pain patient are less sophisticated methods to reproduce the same physiological effects without having to consult a health professional. This allows such a modality to be used as a regular pain-management strategy or one that is employed at specific times of need. In these circumstances patients are active participants in their own healthcare, being able to choose what, when, where and how they should be treated. In this respect they are their own therapist.

With a basic understanding of the therapeutic effects of cutaneous stimulation and a knowledge of safe and simple methods of application the health professional is in a position to empower the patient with some straightforward strategies.

Superficial heating

Numerous modalities are available for warming superficial and deep tissues. Although some, such as short-wave diathermy, are more effective at heating deep tissues, they are not available to the patient. As the focus for this chapter is to highlight strategies that empower the patient, only superficial heating will be discussed.

Physiological effects of superficial heating

A complex set of physiological and systemic changes accompanies any local tissue heating. These can be largely classified into metabolic, haemodynamic, neuromuscular and analgesic effects.

Metabolic effects

Metabolic activity increases with a rise in temperature. With increasing heat an optimal tissue temperature is reached at which metabolic activity is maximally stimulated. Beyond this temperature increasing heat denatures proteins and interferes with metabolic processes. Temperatures above 45°C create so much protein destruction that tissue damage takes place.

Haemodynamic effects

Skin temperature, and to a lesser extent subcutaneous tissue temperature, rise with the application of superficial heating. In order to dissipate the additional heat, and to protect the heated skin, vasodilatation occurs. Little heating occurs in the deeper tissues or more deeply placed joints because the subcutaneous fat insulates them and heat is removed in the increased skin blood flow. There is an increase in blood flow to the skin and superficial tissues but there is a decrease in blood flow to the underlying musculature.

Analgesic effects

There is evidence that local heating of the skin alters cutaneous sensations. Hyperalgesia occurs in the area of the heated region. This may be due to the influence of skin mechanoreceptors on pain modulation (Cervero et al., 1993). This effect does not last long after the cessation of heating. Afferent nerves that are stimulated by heat are believed to have an analgesic effect by acting on the pain-gate mechanism. As superficial heating primarily affects the skin it is assumed that the major pain-relieving effects in the subcutaneous structures are reflex.

Therapeutic effects and indications for treatment

Relief from pain and muscle spasm, improved flexibility, enhanced relaxation and healing are among some of the major therapeutic effects of superficial heating. It is useful to remember that more than one symptom may exist, for example a tense, stiff and painful neck, in the same patient. Often these are interconnected. In the same way several of the effects of superficial heating are interrelated.

Relief of pain

Therapeutic heat is used extensively for pain relief. Several studies have shown that patients with chronic pain rate the use of heat as a pain control strategy highly after analgesia. Not only may superficial heating achieve pain relief by acting on the pain gate but it may also help reduce muscle spasm, contribute to the reduction of joint and soft tissue stiffness and improve relaxation. These factors may all have an effect that helps to reduce pain. Moreover, the increase in blood flow due to heating may reduce ischaemic pain, flush out pain-provoking metabolites and encourage endorphin release.

Heating is largely confined to the superficial tissues but some conduction does occur to the deeper tissues. The decrease in sympathetic nervous system activity, which accompanies superficial heating, is believed to encourage vasodilatation in deeper blood vessels (Michlovitz, 1986). These factors justify the application of superficial heat for such conditions as osteoarthritis of the knee.

Reduction of muscle spasm

Muscle spasm and pain may be interrelated. An increase in pain may cause an increase in spasm resulting in a further increase in pain. The reverse is also true. A reduction in pain may cause a reduction in muscle spasm resulting in further reduction in pain.

Increased flexibility

Superficial heating is used widely in combination with strategies, such as muscle stretching and joint mobilization, to improve flexibility. There are several mechanisms by which superficial heating promotes greater flexibility. Any reduction in pain, as a result of tissue heating, will allow a greater tolerance of joint mobilization and soft tissue stretching. Joint stiffness will also be reduced as a result of heating lowering the fluid viscosity (Wright and Johns, 1961).

Heat can therefore be used prior to exercises designed to stretch muscles, lengthen scars or contractures or mobilize joints. This is particularly useful to the patient who suffers 'morning stiffness' as a result of a chronic joint condition such as rheumatoid arthritis. Where joint stiffness or soft tissue inflexibility contributes to the pain experienced by a patient, reduction of stiffness and inflexibility will result in a reduction in pain.

Relaxation

Superficial heating leads to a reduction in pain and muscle tension. These factors may contribute to the sedative effect observed in patients who have undergone heat treatment. Lehmann and de Lateur (1982) suggested that the sedative effect of superficial heat application might be due to a reflex phenomenon as it had been observed that skin temperatures rise prior to sleep.

Enhanced healing

Therapeutic heating can be applied to a wide range of chronic inflammatory states and post-traumatic conditions including soft tissue lesions and post-surgical healing. Vasodilatation, resulting from superficial heating, will increase the inflow of nutrients, leukocytes and antibodies to the heated area and increase the removal of breakdown products. In addition superficial heating may enhance healing by increasing fluid exchange, metabolic rate and cell activity in the area. Chronic inflammation may be helped by the same mechanisms. Thus superficial heating can be used to enhance healing and reduce inflammation in many subacute and chronic musculoskeletal injuries or conditions.

Table 9.1 Contraindications and precautions for heat treatment

Contraindications	Precautions
Sensory deficiency (altered skin sensations)	Temperature control of heat treatment
Vascular insufficiency (arteriosclerosis)	Pain increases as temperature rises
Ischaemic changes	Patients' understanding of effects of heat therapy – should be confident when applied
Risk of haemorrhage	If too hot can lead to tissue damage and burns
Acute musculoskeletal injury (before bruising occurs)	Not to be used longer than 20–30 minutes
Compromised clotting disfunction	Application of heat therapy with a wet towel against the skin
Pressure of tumour (direct contact to area)	

Methods of application

There are many ways in which superficial heat can be applied to the body:

- The most obvious is the hot water bottle.
- Electrical heating pads and microwave packs are equally effective and convenient.
- Paraffin wax for home use to heat the extremities, particularly the hands. This, however, may be less convenient as it is time-consuming, messy and difficult to use.
- For similar effects the hands, or other parts of the body, can be immersed in a basin or bowl of hot water.
- To capitalize on the relaxation or soporific effects of heat simply taking a hot bath or shower will help. For the creative patient, exercise whilst immersed in water will capitalize not only on the therapeutic effects of superficial heating but also on the buoyancy of the water giving support to the joints.

Summary

Superficial heat application is a simple and effective strategy that patients can use for symptom control. Although the therapeutic effects are only temporary, the patient can use this strategy repeatedly without the need for a health professional and as such it can form part of an ongoing package of self-management. Interestingly, many of the therapeutic effects of heat are also seen in the application of cold therapy.

Cold therapy

Cold therapy is the therapeutic use of local or general body cooling. Whereas superficial heating adds heat energy to the superficial tissues, cooling transfers heat energy away by conduction. Both heat and cold therapy are used to reduce pain and muscle spasm.

Physiological effects of tissue cooling

Cooling the surface of the skin will bring about local changes at that site and systemic changes as the thermoregulating mechanisms of the body are initiated.

Metabolic effects

Metabolic activity decreases with a fall in temperature. As cooling increases, metabolic activity is progressively reduced. Ultimately tissue destruction will occur if the cellular fluid becomes frozen.

Haemodynamic effects

Skin temperature and to a much lesser degree deep tissue temperature drop with the application of superficial cold. In order to diminish heat loss from the skin there is instant vasoconstriction of the cutaneous blood vessels. This vasoconstriction may be replaced by vasodilatation after several minutes, only for vasoconstriction to take place again after about another 15 minutes. This rotation of vasoconstriction and vasodilatation is called the 'hunting reaction' (Lewis, 1930).

Vasoconstriction is thought to occur as an autonomic reflex initiated by stimulation of the thermal receptors of the skin. Cold may also directly affect the arteriole smooth muscle and indirectly affect the precapillary sphincters in order to effect vasoconstriction (Lee and Warren, 1978). Local circulation will also be slowed by increased blood viscosity. Episodic vasodilatation is believed to occur only when the temperature is sufficiently low that prolonged cooling would cause ischaemia and subsequent tissue destruction.

Neuromuscular effects

Initially cooling stimulates cold receptors of muscle and nerve fibres. With reducing temperatures nerve conduction rates continue to fall until conduction ceases. If muscle temperature is reduced reflex activity is lessened. These effects have been shown to continue for a significant amount of time following the application and removal of the cooling medium.

Analgesic effects

Studies have shown that cold therapy is likely to reduce pain perception by acting on the pain-gate mechanism in the same way as other sensory stimuli, such as TENS and acupuncture (Melzack et al., 1980).

Therapeutic effects and indications for treatment

Tissue cooling shares a number of therapeutic effects with heat therapy such as relief from pain and muscle spasm and, in the same way, these are interrelated – a reduction in one will result in a reduction in the other. Additional effects include the reduction of inflammation, effusion, oedema and tissue damage, and improved strength and flexibility.

Relief of pain

Tissue cooling will help reduce local oedema that distorts the tissues stimulating pain nerve endings and slow the release of pain-provoking hormones such as kinins and histamine in response to tissue injury, and hence reduce pain. For these reasons cold therapy is often used in acute trauma such as sports injuries where pain can often be alleviated or even prevented by early application. Pain relief will also come from a reduction in muscle spasm.

Reduction of muscle spasm

Pain and muscle spasm appear to be interdependent. Pain may trigger muscle spasm as a protective mechanism; however, muscle spasm appears to result in pain by causing tissue ischaemia and thus a vicious cycle occurs. As tissue cooling reduces nerve conduction velocities and reflex activity it may effect a reduction in muscle spasm, with a consequential reduction in pain resulting in further reduction in muscle spasm.

Tissue cooling may also be used to reduce muscle spasticity and has good evidence to support its effectiveness. Decreased muscle tone is achieved by lowering the muscle temperature sufficiently to effect a reduction in reflex activity.

Reduction of inflammation, effusion and oedema

Cold therapy is a well-recognized strategy in the management of inflammation, effusion and oedema. Tissue cooling reduces inflammation by impeding the release of histamine and, although this effect is more significant in acute conditions, chronic conditions may be helped by the control of small acute or subacute inflammatory changes that may arise.

Joint and tissue swelling are reduced as a result of vasoconstriction, which reduces blood flow and capillary pressure and slows local metabolism. The addition of compression to cold enhances the control of acute swelling.

Reduction of tissue damage

Superficial heating enhances healing as described in the previous section but tissue cooling may serve to delay healing due to the effects of vasoconstriction and reduced metabolic activity. However, these effects are invaluable in limiting tissue damage due to injury.

A documented sequence of events takes place following an injury:

• Bleeding takes place and plasma is released into the tissues. Cell necrosis takes place over an interval of hours and results in a release of lysins into the area, which provokes local oedema.
• Cell necrosis extends the injury site.
• The early application of cold therapy will limit bleeding and tissue swelling due to vasoconstriction and will lessen the occurrence of secondary cell necrosis by reducing metabolic activity.

Increased flexibility

Tissue cooling, having been shown to modify muscle stretch reflexes, may enhance a stretch programme.

Methods of application

As with the application of heat, patients planning to use cold therapy should understand its therapeutic effects and the precautions required for safe application.

There are several methods of cold application available to a patient:

• Choice may depend on convenience and the body part requiring cooling.
• Ice packs are most commonly used and can be made by folding crushed ice into a damp towel and applying it directly to the skin.
• Equally the crushed ice can be placed into a polythene bag and applied to oiled skin covered by a damp towel.

Table 9.2 Contraindications and precautions for cold therapy

Contraindications	Precautions
Patients suffering hypertension or hypotension – may provoke angina/ coronary heart disease	Sensory deficiency (altered skin sensation)
Raynaud's phenomenon (limb ischaemia)	Patient understanding of possible effects
Buerger's disease (obstruction)	If too cold, ice burns might result
Connective tissue disease (cryoglobulinaemia)	Application of cold therapy with wet towel to skin
Cold urticaria	Skin checking every few minutes, before/after
	Protect skin with oil
	Do not place full weight of limb/body part on ice pack – causes local ischaemia

- A bag of frozen peas is the traditional convenient substitute for both these methods. These methods have been found to be equally effective (De Domenico et al., 1991).
- Disturbing the ice pack while checking the skin promotes lower skin temperatures – the skin will warm the thin layer of water with which it is in contact.
- Commercial cold packs and chemical packs are also available. The former comprises a vinyl bag of fluid that can be cooled in the freezer. This cools the skin more rapidly than traditional ice packs but warms more quickly, providing cooling for approximately 20 minutes.
- Chemical packs rely on the endothermic reaction achieved by mixing two chemicals. They are one-use only packs and therefore may be suitable as a first-aid measure when ice packs are unavailable. Chemical packs do not cool the tissues as effectively as ice packs.
- Ice baths, a mixture of water and ice, may be used and may be useful for cooling the extremities. Increasing the amount of ice and agitating the water will effect more rapid cooling. Ice baths are made more comfortable by alternating the body part in and out of the water.
- Placing a towel in a bath of water and crushed ice, wringing it out and applying it to the body makes an ice towel. Ice towels warm rapidly and

need to be replaced every few minutes but are useful for cooling larger areas and allowing exercises to be executed simultaneously.

- Ice massage can be given by moving a lump of ice, held in a paper towel, in a slow circular manner over the area to be treated. This is effective for pain relief, often within 10 minutes, as the part becomes numb.
- Cold sprays may be useful. These should be sprayed in strokes, from approximately 50 cm, onto the skin at right angles, each spray lasting 5 seconds. This method may cool the skin rapidly but does not last very long.

Summary

It can be seen that cold therapy, like superficial heat, is another straightforward and helpful strategy for independent symptom control.

Massage

Massage is the application of touch or force to soft tissues, usually muscles, tendons or ligaments, without causing movement or change in the position of a joint (Haldeman and Hooper, 1999). Massage is instinctive; when we injure ourselves we rub the part, when we are tense and sore we manipulate and massage the area. This is for good reason as massage is one of the oldest and most advantageous methods of pain relief, which capitalizes on the effect of sensory stimulation on the pain gate. A full explanation of the gate-control theory can be found in Chapter 2.

Physiological effects of massage

The physiological effects of massage can be grouped into three main areas: circulatory, connective tissue and analgesic effects.

Circulatory effects

Moving a hand over the surface of the skin causes friction, which in turn creates heat. The heat stimulates vasodilatation and an increase in tissue permeability. The force of the moving hand on the skin alters pressure in the tissue spaces and vessels. These pressure changes push fluid from the tissue spaces into the vessels and on to the lymph nodes and heart. As a consequence new fluid is drawn into the tissue spaces.

Connective tissue effects

Collagen is remodelled and arranged along the lines of stress in response to mechanical stress. Massage, like functional activity, will place a mechanical stress through the soft tissues by elongating and stretching the fibres. As such, massage will promote remodelling and an increase in tensile strength.

Analgesic effects

Research shows that there is little reliable evidence that massage relieves pain despite the fact that everyone will use it instinctively for that very purpose. Two main explanations have been proposed for the pain relief that people experience. The first is that the sensory stimulation provided by hands on the skin will activate the pain-gate mechanism. The second is that massage will stimulate the production of endorphins although this has yet to be demonstrated.

Therapeutic effects of massage and indications for use

The major therapeutic effects of massage are relief from pain and muscle spasm, improved flexibility and enhanced relaxation. In keeping with the therapeutic effects seen in heat therapy these effects appear interrelated and interdependent.

Relief of pain

Massage may have an indirect effect on the pain by modifying the cause of the pain such as increased muscle tone and reduced soft tissue flexibility. Massage will increase circulation, tissue permeability and fluid exchange. Elimination of excess fluid trapped in the tissues reduces pressure on sensitive nerve endings and may remove pain-provoking waste products and thus reduce pain.

This effect is important both in acute pain states such as delayed-onset muscle soreness where pain and stiffness follows exercise as a result of connective tissue inflammation and in swelling within the muscle, but also in chronic pain states where reduced circulation and fluid exchange will lead to the build-up of metabolites.

Relief of muscle spasm

Muscle spasm occurs, as a protective mechanism, in response to pain. However, muscle spasm itself provokes pain as the excess tone reduces local circulation. As a result metabolites build up which irritate sensory nerve endings and eventually local oedema, soft tissue adhesions and muscle shortening may occur as these symptoms develop into a pathophysiological cycle.

This complex set of events may occur in a number of situations. A normal response to stress is an increase in tone in the muscles of the shoulder girdle.

The posture may change with the upper back and neck being held rigid and the shoulders raised. As the muscles are effectively being over-used they rapidly use their energy supplies and quickly fatigue. The static tension reduces local circulation resulting in a reduced inflow of energy and removal of waste products. Poor posture may occur for reasons other than stress, for example, low mood, poor habits or environmental factors. Whatever the cause inefficient body positioning may lead to the same set of physiological reactions. In a similar fashion muscle tension may develop in response to occupational demands. Most common are those that involve holding a static posture such as that used by typists. In some more than one of these circumstances may exist, for example holding up a book to read while curled up on the sofa.

This 'vicious cycle' of events can be broken by massage, which appears to reduce muscle tone, reduce excess tissue fluid, replenish energy and flush out waste products. Early recognition and intervention may help prevent chronic tension states, and promote muscle balance and postural symmetry.

Increased flexibility

Following injury, accident or surgery, scar tissue is laid down to repair the area. This is deposited in a haphazard arrangement, bridging the gap in the broken fibres and subsequently shortening. Normal functional activity such as active movements will place a stress through the new tissue, which is important to encourage appropriate remodelling.

In the absence of injury, reduced mechanical stress will result in a reduction in flexibility and tensile strength of the soft tissues. Moreover soft tissue adhesions and muscle shortening can occur as a result of a prolonged state of muscle tension.

In all such circumstances massage is useful to provide a mechanical stress, which promotes remodelling along lines of stress thereby encouraging connective tissue to regain normal flexibility, strength and length. Although this may be a useful addition to a programme aimed at the rehabilitation of normal functional movement it is particularly helpful where such a programme is limited by pain or the nature of the injury and its management.

Inflexibility of a small area of soft tissue will have an adverse effect on the overall flexibility of a body part and indeed of the body. Massage may therefore be an important strategy to help regain full flexibility, restore function and prevent reinjury.

Enhanced relaxation

Many patients with chronic pain, anxiety or depression will display unhelpful postures and movement patterns as a result of the physical and emotional effects of their chronic condition. Often the frustration of living with a body that no longer functions as it once did will manifest itself in tension, position and movement.

Massage may help reduce the muscle tension associated with low activity and low mood states and bring about an enhanced state of relaxation. Massage, however, has also been linked to self-esteem in several studies and as such may have a place in contributing to a positive self-image in those patients in chronic pain. Pain and low levels of activity often contribute to poor sleep patterns and massage is reported to effect a better quality and quantity of sleep in such circumstances.

Table 9.3 Contraindications and precautions for using massage

Contraindications	Precautions
Weak fragile tissues (newly healing tissues, diabetes, long-term steroids)	Tissues should be sufficiently robust to withstand massage (mechanical force)
Blood vessels that are weak and damaged	Bacterial and fungal infections (risk of spread)
Poor clotting (haemophilia)	Active infections/malignancies (lymphatic flow = spread)
Deep vein thrombosis – risk of dislodging the clot	
History of cardiac disease	
Newly diagnosed cancer – not to massage over cancer site as blood flow is increased	

Self-massage techniques

To discourage the patient from becoming therapy dependent it is important to teach the skills of self-massage. A patient can then use massage as a strategy when and as often as they choose. Massage should ideally be carried out in a warm, quiet and well-ventilated environment. If the person is cold relaxation will be difficult. Prior to starting massage, consideration should be given to whether the use of a lubricant is appropriate or not. Either powder or oil may be used as a lubricant and will reduce friction of the hands on the skin. This is particularly useful if the skin is fragile to prevent overstretching or if the skin is hairy to prevent pulling on the hairs. However, a lubricant may not allow deeper tissues to be manipulated.

Four techniques from many are described below.

Superficial stroking (effleurage)

This is a gentle movement applied using the whole hand with the fingers together or with the palm to cover a large surface area. The hands, in continuous contact with the skin, conform to the shape of the part being massaged and a smooth, flowing, rhythmical action is used. Light pressure will exert an influence on the superficial tissues and is a useful technique with which to start and finish a massage session or to effect relaxation and identify areas of general tension. Deeper pressure will affect the deeper structures and is usually applied in the direction of venous or lymphatic flow to reduce oedema.

Kneading

This technique differs from stroking as the skin moves with the hands over the subcutaneous tissues rather than the hands moving over the skin. The tissues may be gripped, compressed or wrung. This is a technique often applied to muscles, which can be alternately grasped, lifted and squeezed and released along their length to increase vasodilatation, relaxation and fluid exchange.

Deep massage (frictions)

Several authors have described these techniques. Cyriax (1971) described this as a technique that uses thumb or finger pads to apply deep pressure transversely across the structure being massaged. Wood (1974) also describes deep pressure applied with the finger or thumb tips but directed in a circular rather than transverse motion. In either case the short deep strokes help with the resolution of local oedema and the release of adhesions, which may exist between soft tissue structures as a result of injury, prolonged muscle spasm or postural dysfunction.

Trigger point release

Trigger points are specific spots of hypersensitivity within a muscle complex that can cause referred pain. They may occur as a result of local ischaemia and a prolonged increase in muscle tone. Among the treatments proposed to deactivate these points is deep pressure applied at 90° to the fibres, by finger or thumb pads, held for a minimum of 20 seconds and repeated three to five times (Travell and Simons, 1992). It is advocated that stretching of the muscle involved follows trigger point release. Travell and Simons (1998) suggest that vapo-coolant spray is used prior to stretching.

Summary

Massage may be a useful strategy in the management of chronic pain. However, as its effects are often short-lived it is imperative that this is used as a self-management strategy that the patient can use independently of the health professional. To do otherwise may disempower rather than enable the patient. The use of massage not only is a pain-relieving strategy but can also be a form of loving communication within a relationship. Such a strategy will capitalize on the 'feel-good factor' chemicals thus enhancing pain relief.

Transcutaneous electrical nerve stimulation

Transcutaneous electrical nerve stimulation (TENS) is the application of electrical stimulation to the skin via surface electrodes in order to stimulate nerve fibres, principally for the relief of pain (Walsh, 1997). It is a convenient low-cost machine, which is straightforward and safe for home use by a patient and therefore comprises a useful self-management strategy.

High-frequency TENS

High-frequency (high-frequency/low-intensity) TENS, also known as conventional TENS, is the most commonly used mode of TENS. The stimulation parameters incorporate a low-intensity current (10–30 mA) with a high frequency (above 100 Hz) and a short pulse duration (50–80 μs).

Low-frequency TENS

Low-frequency (low-frequency/high-intensity) TENS, also known as acupuncture-like TENS, incorporates a low frequency (usually 1–4 Hz) with a high intensity (20–50 mA – until muscle contraction is elicited) and a long pulse duration (about 200 μs).

In addition, many TENS units offer the user the choice of continuous, burst and modulated outputs. The continuous and burst outputs are easy to understand. The modulated output provides variation in frequency, pulse duration or amplitude parameters in a cyclical fashion. Manufacturers have included the choice of modulated output to overcome accommodation of nerve fibres and to provide patient comfort. The primary function of TENS is to relieve pain. There are two major mechanisms by which it is suggested TENS achieves this.

Gate-control theory

The gate-control theory of pain proposed by Melzack and Wall in 1965 stated that stimulation of large-diameter (C) fibres could reduce pain perception brought about by activity in the small-diameter (A – types 1 and 2) fibres. This theory acted as a driver for the production of afferent stimulation techniques, most notably TENS. A full explanation of the gate-control theory is given in Chapter 2.

Selective activation of C-fibres requires a low-intensity, high-frequency stimulus with short pulse duration. High-frequency TENS therefore stimulates the A-fibre afferents. The sensation experienced with high-frequency TENS is one of comfortable paraesthesia (a tingling sensation) with no muscle contractions. Analgesia is of relatively rapid onset but tends to be relatively short, typically lasting only for up to a few hours post-treatment. As the C-fibres are stimulated, this mode of TENS achieves analgesia primarily by spinal segmental mechanisms – gating effects.

Endogenous opioid activity

Ascending noiciceptive fibres initiate activity in the periaqueductal grey matter (PAG), an area rich in opioid receptors, causing the release of opioids. In turn the PAG neurons exert an excitatory effect on the rostral ventral medulla (RVM) whose neurons project to the spinal cord and inhibit nociception.

Low-frequency TENS therefore stimulates the nociceptive fibres and small motor fibres. The sensation experienced with low-frequency TENS is one of paraesthesia (a tingling sensation) and muscle contraction (twitching type) with this mode. As muscle contractions occur, additional sensory information is carried from the muscle spindle via muscle afferents. Analgesia is of a relatively longer onset but typically lasts longer than with high-frequency TENS. Naxolone reverses the effects of low-frequency TENS, signifying that the effects may be produced by endogenous opioid receptor activity.

Therapeutic effects and indications for treatment

Some evidence indicates that TENS may be an effective strategy for the management of acute pain. Disappointingly, however, the same cannot be said for the treatment of chronic pain, as evidence is inconsistent in this area. Some of the evidence is outlined in Table 9.4. Table 9.5 highlights the contraindications for the use of TENS and precautions that need to be taken.

Application of TENS

The clinician and client have a number of parameters from which to select: electrode placement, mode of TENS (frequency, intensity, pulse duration) and treatment time.

Table 9.4 Some of the evidence supporting use of TENS in acute and chronic pain*

Acute pain	Chronic pain
Dysmenorrhoea (low abdominal pain felt at/around menstruation) – demonstrated to reduce pain and intensity (Dawood and Ramos, 1990; Milsom et al., 1994)	Effectiveness of TENS for management of chronic pain remains unvalidated
Sim (1991) found significantly less pain at rest, on deep breathing and coughing in TENS and analgesia group for patients following cholecystectomy	Taylor et al. (1981) compared active and placebo TENS in patients with osteoarthritic knee. Difference in pain and medication score between both groups
Systematic review revealed little pain relief in acute post-operative conditions (TENS vs sham TENS and opioids) (Carroll et al., 1996)	TENS useful in neuropathic pain studies for symptom management (Meyler and De Jongste, 1994; Fishbain et al., 1996; Nathan and Wall, 1997)
Effective in treatment of angina. Reduction in myocardial ischaemia (Chauhan et al., 1994)	Leijon and Boivie (1989) – effect of TENS on central neuropathic pain states following stroke – found slight reduction in pain
	Many patients value use of TENS on a long-term basis
	Traditionally used for low back pain – little evidence to support effectiveness
	Although evidence is poor does not mean that it does not work (McQuay and Moore, 1998)

*See Walsh (1997) for more examples.

Treatment time

Initially a brief treatment session will allow the clinician to assess patients and teach them how to use the equipment and will give the patient the chance to experience the sensation. At home patients may then use the TENS in sessions of not less than 30 minutes and as frequently as desired. If low-frequency TENS is being used it is important to warn the patient that where contraction is elicited muscle fatigue might occur. Ideally, a session of TENS will be followed by a period of post-stimulation analgesia.

Table 9.5 Contraindications and precautions for using TENS

Contraindications	Precautions
Epilepsy	Sensory deficiency (altered skin sensation)
Raynaud's phenomenon (limb ischaemia)	Patient understanding of possible effects and ability to place electrodes on painful body parts
Buerger's disease (obstruction)	Do not use over sore or broken skin – can cause burns
Connective tissue disease (cryoglobulinaemia)	Can cause skin irritation
Pacemaker	Warn against using TENS while using machinery and driving
First trimester of pregnancy – can cause premature labour if put over pregnant uterus	Do not wear in bath or shower – can cause burns
Not to be placed on carotid area (front of neck or larynx) and eyes	Do not use if equipment appears unsafe

Summary

Transcutaneous electrical nerve stimulation, having mixed reviews, may be a useful treatment strategy for the management of acute pain. In chronic pain, evidence for efficacy is even less clear. It is, however, worth noting that a proportion of patients with chronic pain will find TENS useful on a long-term basis as part of an overall pain-management strategy. As TENS is an independently used, cost-effective, convenient modality, which has few side effects, it remains worthy of attention in this group of patients.

Conclusion

Before using any of the strategies discussed in this chapter with a patient a thorough assessment should be made. This will allow the clinician the basis from which to reason how a strategy may be helpful.

Ice, massage and TENS have been compared as treatments for low back pain. Melzack et al. (1980) compared the application of TENS and ice massage over acupuncture points in chronic low back pain patients. They found a significant reduction in McGill Pain Scores in the ice massage group. In a comparison of TENS with mechanical massage delivered via four suction cups Melzack et al. (1983) reported greater pain relief in the TENS group coupled with a significant increase in straight leg raise.

However, often more than one strategy may be useful and this will allow the patient to choose or to explore the value of combination treatment. For example, muscle spasm occurring as a result of back pain may be treated with heat, which promotes relaxation and stimulates vasodilatation. Equally, ice will produce a similar result by cooling the muscle and reducing spindle activity.

In addition it is useful to consider how any of the self-treatment strategies may enhance the effect of other pain-management or rehabilitation strategies. For example, Friedland (1955) reports that the effectiveness of a joint mobilization or soft tissue-stretching programme may be enhanced by the use of heat, which will reduce pain and increase extensibility, making such a programme less painful and more effective. Cold therapy may exert an influence on the motor neuron pool resulting in an increase in strength and, as previously highlighted, massage is an obvious addition to a programme designed to increase flexibility. TENS, via a reduction in pain, may allow a patient to participate more fully in a fitness programme such as a walking programme. With such a battery of useful and validated strategies the clinician is in a strong position to empower pain patients to manage their pain.

References

Carroll D, Tramer M, McQuay H et al. (1996) Randomisation is important in studies with pain outcomes: systematic review of transcutaneous electrical nerve stimulation in acute post-operative pain. British Journal of Anaesthesia 77: 798–803.

Cervero F, Gilbert R, Hammond RGE et al. (1993) Development of secondary hyperalgesia following non-painful thermal stimulation of the skin: a psychophysical study in man. Pain 54: 181–9.

Chauhan A, Mullins PA, Thuraisingham SI et al. (1994) Effect of transcutaneous electrical nerve stimulation on coronary blood flow. Circulation 2: 694–702.

Cyriax J (1971) Textbook of Orthopaedic Medicine, Diagnosis of Soft Tissue Lesions Vol 1, 6th edn. London: Baillière Tindall.

Dawood MY, Ramos J (1990) Transcutaneous electrical nerve stimulation (TENS) for the treatment of primary dysmenorrhea: a randomized cross-over comparison with placebo TENS and ibuprofen. Obstetrics and Gynecology 75: 656–60.

De Domenico G, Cotton S, Devereux D et al. (1991) Skin temperature changes with different methods of cryotherapy. WCPT, 11th International Congress Proceedings. Book II. London: World Confederation for Physical Therapy, pp. 606–8.

Fishbain DA, Chabal C, Abbott A et al. (1996) Transcutaneous electrical nerve stimulation (TENS) treatment outcome in long term users. Clinical Journal of Pain 12(3): 210–14.

Friedland F (1955) Ultrasonic therapy in rheumatic diseases. American Journal of Physical Medicine 34(2): 379–85.

Haldeman S, Hooper PD (1999) Mobilisation, manipulation, massage and exercise for the relief of musculoskeletal pain. In Wall PD, Melzack R (eds) Textbook of Pain, 4th edn. Edinburgh: Churchill Livingstone.

Lee JM, Warren MP, Mason SM (1978) Effects of ice on nerve conduction velocity. Physiotherapy 64: 2–6.

Lehmann JF, de Lateur BJ (1982). Therapeutic heat. In Lehmann JF (ed.) Therapeutic Heat and Cold. Physical Medicine Library, Vol 2. Baltimore, MD: Lippincott, Williams & Wilkins, pp. 404–562.

Leijon G, Boivie J (1989) Central post stroke pain – the effect of high and low frequency TENS. Pain 38: 187–91.

Lewis T (1930) Observation upon the reactions of the reactions of the vessels of the human skin to cold. Heart 15: 177–208.

McQuay HJ, Moore RA (1998) Transcutaneous electrical nerve stimulation (TENS) in chronic pain. In McQuay HJ, Moore RA (eds) An Evidenced-based Resource for Pain Relief. Oxford: Oxford University Press.

Melzack R (1994) Folk medicine and the sensory modulation of pain. In Wall PD, Melzack R (eds) Textbook of Pain, 3rd edn. Edinburgh: Churchill Livingstone, p. 1210.

Melzack R, Wall PD (1965) Pain mechanisms: a new theory. Science 150: 971–9.

Melzack R, Jeans ME, Stratford JG et al. (1980) Ice massage and transcutaneous electrical stimulation: comparison of treatment for low back-pain. Pain 9: 209–17.

Melzack R, Vetere P, Finch L (1983) Transcutaneous electrical nerve stimulation for low back pain. Physical Therapy 63: 489–93.

Meyler WJ, De Jongste MJL (1994) Clinical evaluation of pain treatment with electro-stimulation: a study on TENS in patients with different pain syndromes. Clinical Journal of Pain 10: 22–7.

Michlovitz SL (1986) Biophysical principles of heating and superficial heat agents. In Michlovitz SL (ed.) Thermal Agents in Rehabilitation. Philadelphia, PA: Davis, pp. 99–118.

Milsom I, Hedner N, Mannheimer C (1994) A comparative study of the effect of high-intensity transcutaneous nerve stimulation and oral naproxen on intrauterine pressure and menstrual pain. American Journal of Obstetrics and Gynecology 1: 123–9.

Nathan PW, Wall PD (1974) Treatment of post-herpetic neuralgia by prolonged electric stimulation. British Medical Journal 3: 645–7.

Sim DT (1991) Effectiveness of transcutaneous electrical nerve stimulation following cholescystectomy. Physiotherapy 77: 715–22.

Taylor P, Hallett M, Flaherty L (1981) Treatment of osteoarthritis of the knee with transcutaneous electrical nerve stimulation. Pain 11: 233–40.

Travell JG, Simons DG (1998) Myofascial Pain and Dysfunction. The Trigger Point Manual, Vol. II. Baltimore, MD: Lippincott, Williams & Wilkins.

Walsh DM (1997) TENS Clinical Applications and Related Theory. Edinburgh: Churchill Livingstone.

Wood ED (1974) Beard's Massage Principles and Techniques. Philadelphia, PA: WB Saunders.

Wright W, Johns, RJ (1961) Quantitative and qualitative analysis of joint stiffness in normal subjects and in patients with connective tissue diseases. Annals of Rheumatic Diseases 20: 36–46.

CHAPTER TEN

Pharmacological management

PETER CROOT

Aim

To review the use of drugs or medicines that have pain-relieving properties.

Objectives

At the end of the chapter the reader will have an understanding of the following:

- Pharmacokinetics – how our body handles medicines. This process commences with *absorption* of the medicine into the body, followed by *distribution* of the medicine around the body including transport to its site(s) of action, and then the body processes medicines to *eliminate* them by *excretion*.
- Pharmacodynamics – how medicines affect our body. A brief overview of how medicines interact with drug receptors will be provided.

Definitions

A dictionary definition of *pharmacology* is 'the science of the action of drugs on the body'. The word 'drugs' is often associated with illicit or recreational use of therapeutic substances, so this chapter will use the term 'medicines' to describe pain-killers.

Pharmacokinetic processes – absorption

Medicines need to transfer from the pharmaceutical formulation administered – for example, tablet, capsule or skin patch – to the blood capillaries,

230

which then distribute the medicine around the body. There are a number of processes involved in absorption but the primary movement of molecules of the medicine is by passive diffusion down a concentration gradient. This applies to medicines absorbed from the intestine, skin and mucous membranes.

Molecules move from an area of high concentration, such as the lumen of the small intestine when a tablet breaks down to release its contents, to an area of lower concentration, commonly the blood flowing through the intestinal wall. Depending on the fat solubility of the molecules they will move down the concentration gradient from the lumen to the blood capillaries. A further factor is the surface area for absorption. The prime absorptive area for many medicines taken by mouth is the jejunal region of the small intestine where the villi provide a large area for absorption. Many medicines are formulated to ensure that they are released in the small intestine and have good fat solubility to aid the absorption down the concentration gradient. Moreover, pharmaceutical formulations can be engineered to provide the following:

- Enteric coatings (EC) on tablets to avoid breakdown of the medicine by gastric acid.
- Modified-release (MR) mechanisms that prolong the absorption of the medicine, so extending its duration of action.
- Prodrugs, which use metabolic processes in the body to convert inactive substances into active medicine.
- Patches for skin application providing transdermal delivery of a medicine.

Pharmacokinetic processes – distribution

Once molecules of a medicine have been absorbed into the bloodstream they must then be circulated to the site of the action in sufficient concentration for the medicine to work. The rate at which a medicine reaches the required part of the body depends on the rate and volume of blood flow to that area of the body. Tissues in organs such as brain, heart, kidneys and lungs that have a good blood supply achieve effective concentrations of medicines easily and quickly, but other factors determine if effective concentrations are maintained at the site of action. These include the extent of binding of molecules to receptors at the site of action, the frequency of dosing, and the rate of removal of the medicine from the bloodstream by metabolic and elimination processes.

Pharmacokinetic processes – elimination

The body has very effective methods for inactivating medicines and removing (excreting) them, to ensure that we do not poison ourselves. For medicines to work they generally have to be soluble in fat (lipid). Water-soluble medicines are easier to excrete as they can be extracted from the blood circulation by the kidneys and passed out in the urine. The liver is able to make small modifications to the molecular structure that change it from being lipid soluble to water soluble. This process is known as metabolization. Many different types of enzymes contained in the liver undertake these chemical modifications. Some can take place in other body tissues. The new molecules produced by the enzymatic processes are called metabolites. Many are inactive, in that they no longer have a pharmacological effect, but some do have a therapeutic effect and are therefore known as active metabolites.

Some metabolites produced by these initial or phase 1 metabolic processes are still not sufficiently water soluble to be eliminated from the body. They undergo further or phase 2 metabolism involving the attachment of another molecule to create a much a larger molecule with better water solubility that can be excreted into urine or bile.

Morphine is broken down to many metabolites. One common metabolite is morphine-6-glucuronide created by the attachment, known as conjugation, of a glucuronide molecule to morphine. This compound is an active metabolite, being more potent than morphine. It is excreted in the urine so in renal impairment it can accumulate in the blood, leading to a prolonged period of action.

Pharmacokinetic processes – excretion

The kidneys are the most important organs for removing medicines and their metabolites from the body. Where renal function is decreased, as in the elderly, medicines excretion is significantly reduced. This requires either the use of *smaller* doses or the use of *standard* doses but with a longer time interval between doses.

Excretion into the bile is an important mechanism for the excretion of some medicines, but this pathway is less efficient than the renal route. Biliary excretion does assume greater significance where there is kidney impairment.

Some medicines are excreted into breast milk and, although this is not a significant route of excretion, it can be harmful to the breast-feeding infant. Amitriptyline, for example, is excreted into breast milk. It does not cause long-term harm to the infant but it may cause undesirable sedation.

Pharmacodynamics – receptor function

Once molecules of a medicine have been absorbed and distributed to their site of action they must trigger a therapeutic response before being eliminated from the body. This most frequently involves interacting with a receptor. A variety of receptors is present on the surface of most cells. Cell receptors recognize certain chemicals whose molecules are of a structure that fits into the receptor, rather like two compatible pieces of a jigsaw fitting together. Once a receptor recognizes a compatible molecule, it binds with it by a firm but reversible chemical bond. The process of chemical binding causes a change in the shape of the receptor protein, which in turn results in a signalling process. With analgesics the signalling might result in the slowing of the electrical impulses within nerves. Many medicines mimic or impair the actions of natural chemicals in the body. The body produces its own natural opioid (morphine-like) substances. The receptors that can respond to these can be stimulated by medicines that are opioid agonists, such as morphine.

Agonists are medicines that initiate a response when they bind with the receptor. *Antagonists* are medicines that bind to the receptor site without causing a response. They prevent natural agonists binding to the receptor, and are often known as receptor blockers. Beta blockers are an example.

There is enormous variation in receptor types and some medicines can have both agonist and antagonist properties. The analgesic buprenorphine is a good example.

Once a receptor has been triggered, how long does the response last? In many instances it is only a matter of milliseconds as the signal molecule is removed from the receptor by enzyme breakdown. Consequently a continuous supply of molecules must be available to the site of action to maintain a continuous response.

Routes of administration of medicines

By mouth

Taking medicines by mouth is the easiest method of administering medicines for most patients. The majority of adults can swallow tablets and capsules. These are designed to break up in the stomach and small intestine. The acid conditions of the stomach can destroy some medicines. This can be overcome by using an enteric coat, which only breaks up in the less acid environment of the small intestine, or a modified release delivery system. Modified-release systems (also referred to as controlled release and slow release) are used to prolong the time period for which the medicine is active.

Medicines absorbed from the stomach and small intestine are taken directly to the liver by the portal circulation. The liver rapidly metabolizes some medicines such that much smaller amounts of active medicine reach the main or systemic blood circulation of the body. This is known as 'first-pass elimination'. If it is a problem it can normally be overcome by administering higher doses.

Sublingual (dissolving a tablet or using a spray under the tongue) and buccal (dissolving a tablet against the gum, usually of the upper jaw) preparations avoid the liver first-pass effect. These routes of administration are an effective way of taking glyceryl trinitrate for anginal pain but are not commonly used in the management of chronic pain.

By rectum

The rectal mucosa provides a good but erratic surface for the absorption of medicine. Medicines are formulated as suppositories or rectal solutions. This method of medicine delivery is not popular with patients and tends to be reserved for short-term management. Non-steroidal anti-inflammatories, such as diclofenac, and some opioids, such as oxycodone, are available in suppository formulations. The rectal route is of limited use in chronic pain management.

Topical

Delivering medicines through the skin is generally the function of messy creams and ointments. Absorption from such formulations is unpredictable, as is movement of medicines through the various skin layers to blood capillaries. The incorporation of medicines into patches, affixed on the skin and which slowly release the medicine, has been a significant pharmaceutical development. Patches are popular with patients and carers. The small doses used can have a therapeutic effect, often with fewer side effects than if the medicine was taken by mouth. The short-acting opioid fentanyl is available in a skin patch that releases the medication for up to 72 hours. Local skin reactions to the material or adhesive of the patches have been reported.

Parenteral

Injectable routes have few uses in the management of chronic pain. A later section describes the intrathecal route – a highly specialized method of medicine delivery suitable for a few patients.

Analgesics and strategies for use

Analgesic use in chronic pain is best based on a common stepwise approach, or ladder. The World Health Organization (WHO) first set out their ladder in 1986 (Figure 10.1). They recognized that pain was an important but neglected public health issue in both developed and developing countries. The aim of widely publicizing the ladder was to educate healthcare professionals throughout the world to use a few effective and relatively inexpensive medicines well and administer them by mouth on a regular basis and according to the individual needs of each patient.

The WHO ladder is a guide to the appropriate use of analgesics in the management of acute and chronic pain. Evaluation of the use of analgesics in cancer pain in accordance with WHO guidance demonstrates that 80% of patients experience pain relief. In the majority the quality of pain relief will be good. However, both the quality and extent of the pain relief are dependent on the analgesics being used correctly. The clinical and pharmaceutical principles to be adhered to in all circumstances when using medicines are:

- right medicine;
- right dose;
- right route;
- right time.

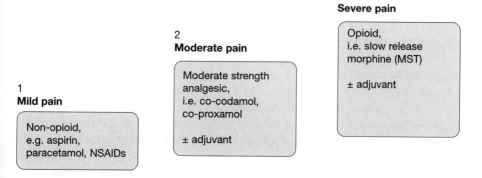

Figure 10.1 World Health Organization analgesic ladder in acute and chronic pain.

Step one – mild pain (Table 10.1)

This involves the use of non-opioids – aspirin, paracetamol, non-steroidal anti-inflammatory drugs (NSAIDs) – with or without the use of adjuvants.

Aspirin

Although it is an effective analgesic, the use of aspirin for this purpose is declining in favour of newer NSAIDs that are better tolerated and easier to take. Aspirin (acetylsalicylic acid) is increasingly being used at low doses for its antiplatelet properties. There is evidence that the cardioprotective effect of low-dose aspirin (75–150 mg once daily) is reduced by concurrent use of ibuprofen, and possibly other NSAIDs.

Aspirin tablets 300 mg enteric coated

The coating is designed to prevent breakdown of the tablet in the stomach and reduce gastric irritation. It breaks up to release the aspirin in the less acidic environment of the small intestine. This delays the onset of action. Enteric-coated tablets are therefore not suitable for single-dose use in acute pain but their prolonged effect may be useful for chronic and night-time pain.

Any retailer can sell aspirin as a general sales list (GSL) medicine. Larger packs can be purchased from registered pharmacies as pharmacy-only (P) medicines.

Individual case reports suggest that lotion formulations of aspirin applied to the skin can be more effective than oral aspirin in the management of postherpetic neuralgia pain. Specialist pharmaceutical units, which supply an unlicensed special against a medical practitioner's prescription, can manufacture this.

Drug interactions occur with the following:

- Anticoagulants – warfarin, nicoumalone. There is an increased risk of bleeding due to the antiplatelet effect of aspirin. It should be avoided in anticoagulated patients.
- Anti-epileptics – phenytoin, valproate. Aspirin can enhance their effects. Regular dosing of aspirin in patients taking one or both of these anti-epileptics is acceptable. 'When required' (p.r.n.) dosing must be avoided as this will cause variation in anti-epileptic blood levels making seizure control difficult.
- Other analgesics. Administration of corticosteroids with aspirin increases the risks of side effects, particularly gastrointestinal bleeding and ulceration.

Paracetamol (acetaminophen)

Due to the lack of platelet inhibition or adverse gastrointestinal effects, this drug is preferable to aspirin in patients who receive oral anticoagulants, have coagulation disorders, or have a history of peptic ulcer disease.

Table 10.1 Step one – mild pain

Drug	Uses	Doses (adult dose)	Frequency	Side effects	Formulation
Aspirin	Colds, menstrual pains, headaches, joints, muscular aches	300–900mg (max 4 g in 24 hours)	4–6 hourly	Nausea and vomiting, gastric bleeding/ulceration – high doses for analgesia should be avoided in high-risk patients. Asthma – can make it worse. Not suitable for children under 16 years	Tablets 300 mg. Enteric coated 300 mg. Suppositories 150 mg, 300 mg. Topical – special order only
Paracetamol	Minor non-inflammatory conditions, pyrexia	500–1000 (1 g) Maximum 4 g in 24 hours	4–6 hourly	Rare. Can get rashes. LIVER DAMAGE if overdose	Tablets 500 mg. Dispersible 500 mg. Solution/suspension 120 mg in 5 ml, 250 mg in 5 ml (available for use in nasogastric or gastrostomy feeding tubes). Suppositories – 500 mg
NSAIDs (ibuprofen)	Rheumatoid arthritis, osteoarthritis, gout, moderate headache, menstrual pain, soft tissue injuries, after surgery	200–400 mg. Maximum 600 mg four times/day or 800 mg three times/day (2.4 g/day max)	8 hourly (see dosing for others)	Nausea/vomiting. Heartburn/indigestion	Tablets – 200 mg, 400 mg, 600 mg. Sustained-release capsules – 300 mg (twice daily administration). Modified release 600 mg (once a day administration). Oral suspension – 100 mg in 5 ml
Diclofenac	Pain and inflammatory diseases, musculoskeletal disorders, acute gout, postoperative pain	75–150 mg a day	Divided into two or three doses	Varies in severity and frequency. Gastrointestinal damage (see BNF for full list)	Tablets – 25 mg, 50 mg. Dispersible 50 mg. Modified release capsules /tablets – 75 mg, 100 mg. Suppositories – 12.5 mg, 25 mg, 50 mg
Celecoxib	As above, high-risk patients using NICE guidelines	100 mg – 200 mg	12 hourly	See BNF	Tablets 100 mg, 200 mg
Rofecoxib	As above	12.5–25 mg (up to 50 mg once a day for acute pain and dysmenhorrhoea)	24 hourly	See BNF	Tablets – 12.5 mg, 25 mg. Suspension – 12.5 mg/5 ml, 25 mg/5 ml

BNF, British National Formulary; NICE, National Institute for Clinical Excellence; NSAIDs, non-steroidal anti-inflammatory drugs.

Small quantities of paracetamol tablets can be purchased as a GSL medicine. Larger packs can be purchased as P medicines. Suppositories can be purchased from registered pharmacies.

Overdose of paracetamol can cause irreversible liver damage, with a toxic metabolite sometimes also causing kidney damage. Paracetamol should be used cautiously in patients with known significant liver damage and patients with alcohol dependence.

Dispersible preparations of paracetamol can contain up to 400 mg sodium per tablet. High doses of the dispersible tablets should be avoided in patients with conditions for which excessive salt intake is unwise, such as hypertension, coronary heart disease, oedema and renal failure.

Prolonged regular use of paracetamol can enhance the effect of warfarin. This should not cause clinical problems if patients have their blood clotting time monitored regularly.

Non-steroidal anti-inflammatory drugs

This is a large group of medicines that have been developed ever since the anti-inflammatory and pain-killing properties of aspirin were discovered. They have become an important element in the management of chronic pain. They are versatile in terms of their routes of administration and differences in potency. A wide range of side effects that can restrict or prevent their use in many patients tempers this versatility.

Most comparisons of NSAIDs are single-dose studies in acute pain; they are valid for the management of chronic pain. An oral dose of ibuprofen 400 mg reduces pain by 50% in one out of two postoperative patients, whereas for paracetamol it is one out of four patients. Ibuprofen is one of the weaker NSAIDs, whereas diclofenac has slightly greater anti-inflammatory activity. There is considerable variation in individual patient response so that a patient who does not find one NSAID effective may respond to another.

Unfortunately as the potency increases so does the extent of gastric bleeding with chronic use. Gastric bleeding induced by NSAIDs is lowest with ibuprofen. Other side effects such as dizziness and drowsiness increase disproportionately with increases in dose. NSAIDs, and aspirin and paracetamol, have a ceiling effect whereby above a certain dose no increase in pharmacological effect is seen.

Celecoxib and rofecoxib are examples of newer NSAIDs known as COX-2 inhibitors. COX is cyclo-oxygenase, an enzyme involved in the production of prostaglandins. The enzyme exists in two forms. COX-1 is always present in various body tissues and is not involved in pain or inflammation. The COX-2 enzyme only appears in damaged tissues shortly after injury and results in the production of inflammatory prostaglandins. The theory is that COX-2-specific NSAIDs inhibit the formation of the inflammatory prostaglandins but do not inhibit the activity of COX-1 in producing the beneficial prostaglandins in tissues such as the stomach and small intestine. COX-2 inhibitors have demonstrated fewer gastrointestinal side effects than older NSAIDs. They can be useful but still must be used cautiously in:

- patients who have previously suffered gastric problems with standard NSAIDs;
- other patients at high risk of developing serious gastrointestinal side effects such as the elderly;
- patients taking other medicines that can adversely affect the gut.

Refer to the current edition of the *British National Formulary* (BNF) or www.bnf.org for details of NSAIDS not listed here.

Any retailer can sell small quantities of ibuprofen 200 mg tablets. Larger quantities of 200 mg and 400 mg tablets and ibuprofen oral suspension can be purchased as P medicines. All other ibuprofen preparations are available on prescription only.

All diclofenac preparations (except those for topical use) are available only on prescription. Celecoxib and rofecoxib are available only on prescription.

There are drug interactions with angiotensin-converting enzyme (ACE) inhibitors and angiotensin II antagonists – NSAIDs can inhibit the blood pressure-lowering effect of medicines such as enalapril and candesartan. There is an increased risk of developing hyperkalaemia.

The use of two NSAIDs together, including aspirin, is best avoided as the likelihood of side effects increases.

Non-steroidal anti-inflammatory drugs can increase the risk of convulsions associated with quinolones such as ciprofloxacin.

The anticoagulant effect of warfarin can be increased by many NSAIDs. This does not cause clinical problems if the NSAIDs are used regularly and the patient's blood clotting time is regularly monitored. The possible interaction becomes significant if there is irregular use of an NSAID.

With regard to antidepressants, there is an increased risk of bleeding in patients taking selective serotonin reuptake inhibitors (SSRIs) such as fluoxetine and paroxetine.

There is an increased probability of the kidney-damaging effects of NSAIDs occurring in patients also receiving diuretics.

The rate of elimination through the kidneys of lithium is reduced by many NSAIDs. Lithium blood levels should be closely monitored when treatment with NSAIDs is commenced and finished.

Step two – moderate pain (Table 10.2)

Weak opioid – used with or without a non-opioid

Weak opioids include codeine, dihydrocodeine and dextropropoxyphene. They are normally administered with aspirin, paracetamol or an NSAID. Paracetamol features in the majority of combinations. Full-dose combinations are required. There is little to be gained from using small doses with paracetamol or from switching from one weak opioid to another.

Codeine

Codeine is an effective opioid analgesic for the relief of mild-to-moderate pain. Its chemical structure is similar to morphine and the liver converts approximately 10% of administered codeine to morphine. The duration of codeine's analgesic effect is around 3 hours. It is also used as a cough suppressant, and its constipating properties are put to good use as an antidiarrhoeal agent.

When this centrally acting analgesic is combined with peripherally acting paracetamol the resultant analgesia is similar to that of small doses of morphine. Small doses of codeine in combination with full doses of paracetamol are inadequate; full doses of both are much more effective. This has been demonstrated by a Bandolier review of studies of paracetamol with codeine in postoperative pain (see the Oxford Pain Internet site at www.jr2.ox.uk/bandolier/booth/painpag/). The standard combination is codeine 60 mg and paracetamol 1000 mg taken every 4–6 hours with a maximum of four doses in 24 hours.

Codeine phosphate injection is sometimes used as an intramuscular analgesic in head injury patients as it is considered to be less sedating than morphine. However, it is a weaker opioid analgesic so trauma patients with head injury are denied the strong analgesia that their injuries may warrant.

Dihydrocodeine

Dihydrocodeine is the product of a slight modification to the codeine molecule and has comparable properties. It is used in similar doses although it is slightly more potent than codeine. It has a shorter duration of action, a factor that limits its usefulness in chronic pain.

Dihydrocodeine is licensed for administration by deep subcutaneous and intramuscular injection. Its use is popular in some hospital accident and emergency units for trauma patients. Its shorter duration of action and lower degree of sedation than morphine can speed the discharge of patients but these possible benefits have to be counterbalanced by its weaker analgesic potency.

Table 10.2 Step two – moderate pain

Drug	Uses	Doses (adult dose)	Frequency	Side effects	Formulation
Codeine phosphate	Mild-to-moderate pain	30–60 mg	4 hourly	Nausea/vomiting, constipation, drowsiness (see BNF for full list)	Tablets – 15 mg, 30 mg, 60 mg Suspension – 25 mg/5 ml Injection – 60 mg/ml
Dihydrocodeine	As above	30 mg	4–6 hourly	As above	Tablets – 30 mg, 40 mg Modified release – 60 mg Oral solution – 10 mg/5 ml Injection – 50 mg/ml
Dextropropoxyphene (in co-proxamol)	As above	(Dextropropoxyphene 32.5 mg/paracetamol 325 mg) Two tablets	6–8 hourly	As above	Tablets – 32.5 mg/325 mg
Tramadol	As above	50–100 mg. Max dose 400 mg in 24 hours	4 hourly	As above	Capsules – 50 mg Soluble tablets – 50 mg Modified release capsules/tablets – 50 mg, 75 mg, 100 mg, 150 mg, 200 mg, 300 mg, 400 mg

BNF, British National Formulary.

Dextropropoxyphene

This morphine derivative is commonly prescribed in association with paracetamol as the combination product co-proxamol. Despite its widespread use, particularly in the elderly with chronic pain associated with arthritic conditions, there is little evidence to support its use. Users with liver or kidney impairment are at risk of toxic effects, and in overdose it is exceedingly dangerous with cardiac conduction problems caused by dextropropoxyphene adding to the major problems arising from paracetamol overdose.

Tramadol

Tramadol is a weak stimulator of opioid receptors. It also has some effects on serotonin release and norepinephrine (noradrenaline) reuptake. In acute pain it has been shown to be as effective as paracetamol but nowhere near as effective as paracetamol and codeine combinations.

It has been marketed as an intermediate step between the step two co-analgesics for moderate pain and step three morphine and other opioids for severe pain. Although it has less respiratory depressant effects than morphine it does not have its analgesic power, so that patients who really require a strong opioid may be deprived of one. In chronic pain it is often prescribed together with a co-analgesic such as co-codamol, leading to additive side effects, particularly somnolence when used in the elderly. At high doses it can accumulate, increasing the risk of seizures.

For a list of preparations see Table 10.2. Refer to the current edition of the *British National Formulary* or www.bnf.org for details of those not listed.

All are prescription-only medicines. Full controlled drug regulations (Misuse of Drugs Act 1971) apply to the injection. Travellers needing to take codeine phosphate preparations abroad may require a doctor's letter explaining why they are necessary.

Dextropropoxyphene is available only in combination with paracetamol as co-proxamol (contains dextropropoxyphene hydrochloride 32.5 mg with paracetamol 325 mg). Co-proxamol tablets are available only on prescription.

Some modified-release preparations of tramadol are intended for *twice* a day dosing, others for *once* a day dosing only. All tramadol preparations are available only on prescription. Convulsions can occur, especially if the maximum daily dose is exceeded

Step three – severe pain

Strong opioids used with or without a non-opioid (Table 10.3)

The use of morphine (Table 10.4) or other strong opioid analgesics is

Table 10.3 Step three – severe pain

Drug	Uses	Doses (adult dose)	Frequency	Side effects	Formulation
Morphine	Severe pain	Titrated to patients' needs	Immediate release – 4 hourly Modified release – 12 hourly 24 hourly	Nausea, vomiting, constipation and drowsiness, with higher doses capable of inducing hypotension in addition to respiratory depression	Immediate release – 10 mg, 20 mg, 50 mg Modified-release capsules and tablets – strengths from 5 mg up to 200 mg Morphine sulphate oral solution 10 mg/5 ml, 100 mg /5 ml
Diamorphine (heroin)	As above	Titrated to patients' needs	Titrated to patients' needs	As above	Injection preparation only Ampoules of freeze-dried powder requiring reconstitution with water for injections or with 0.9% sodium chloride 10 mg, 30 mg, 100 mg, 500 mg strengths.
Oxycodone	As above Palliative care	Titrated to patients' needs	Immediate release – 4 hourly Modified release – 12 hourly Injection/infusion	As above	Capsules – 5 mg, 10 mg, 20 mg immediate release Oral solutions – 5 mg in 5 ml, 10 mg in 1 ml – 4–6 hourly dosing Modified release – 5 mg, 10 mg, 20 mg, 40 mg, 80 mg Injection or infusion – 10 mg in 1 ml

sometimes necessary in the management of chronic pain. For a small number of patients opioids are the only effective pain relievers (Simpson, 2004).

Despite their effectiveness the use of opioids in non-cancer pain is considered controversial. There is a misconception that opioids are addictive and shorten life (Table 10.5). Only by educating the public and health professionals that, when properly used, morphine and related medicines are safe, effective and do not affect life expectancy, will these fears be allayed. We all have a duty to ensure that patients in pain are not denied a treatment that works, because of misguided beliefs and attitudes. Unfortunately the word 'morphine' does frighten some doctors, patients and carers and many associate it solely with use in the last stages of life. Clear explanations of the reasons for its use, the possible side effects and the strategies available to minimize them are essential for full concordance between prescriber and patient.

Opioids work by binding to opioid receptors that are found throughout the central and peripheral nervous systems. A number of different opioid receptors have been discovered. These include μ (mu), κ (kappa) and δ (delta). The clinical significance of these different receptors and the variation in activity of individual opioids interacting with them is unclear. Morphine is an opioid agonist in that it solely stimulates the receptors. Other opioids such as buprenorphine have both agonist (positive) and antagonist (negative) properties. If buprenorphine is given to patients already receiving morphine or another opioid, it may precipitate opioid withdrawal symptoms.

Dose titration of opioids

Literature reviews published on the Oxford Pain website show (see Further Reading) that opioids provide over 60% of users with good or moderate pain relief. In some chronic pain conditions, often where the nervous system is damaged, the response to opioids is poor. The correct way to use opioids is to titrate the doses administered to the degree of pain, with the aim being to achieve pain relief. If the patient still complains of pain after the dose given has been fully absorbed then it is safe to give another dose. The next dose may be smaller than the first.

If pain control is still not achieved then further doses can be given. This principle of titration avoids the respiratory depression associated with opioids that continues to be a concern of many healthcare workers. Opioids can slow and sometimes stop breathing when given to patients who are not in pain, or when larger doses than necessary are administered. By tailoring doses to the degree of pain experienced respiratory depression is minimized. For opioids, the ceiling effect seen with other classes of analgesics is not evident. There are no maximum doses to be adhered to if the titration principle is followed.

Table 10.4 Adverse effects of morphine

Central nervous system	Respiratory	Cardiovascular	Gastrointestinal	Eyes	Skin
Sedation and euphoria have previously been described. Muscular rigidity can occur with high doses, which can occasionally produce convulsions. A slight decrease in body temperature may be seen. Morphine can affect a number of hormones, leading to a reduction in blood concentrations of cortisol and testosterone, causing decreased libido, and an increase in circulating prolactin. Nausea and vomiting is caused by morphine stimulating the chemoreceptor trigger zone. It is more common in ambulant patients than those confined to bed	The respiratory rate is reduced. It has an antitussive effect, although codeine is the preferred cough suppressant	Morphine lowers blood pressure, which is most commonly seen when patients stand up. It may reduce heart rate and relaxes both arterial and venous blood vessels	Morphine relaxes smooth muscle, slowing down gastrointestinal transit. This in turn increases water absorption from the colon leading to constipation	Pupillary constriction occurs. Pinpoint pupils are a characteristic feature of morphine overdose	Peripheral vasodilatation occurs, leading to flushing of the face, neck and upper chest. This may be due to histamine release, which could account for the urticaria sometimes seen at the site of injection. Itching experienced by some patients receiving epidural or intraspinal morphine can be reversed by small doses of naloxone

Table 10.5 Safety of opioids in chronic pain – common misconceptions

Problem	Misconception	Reality
Addiction	Patients develop compulsive reliance on opioids that might adversely affect one or more of the following: • physical health • psychological health • social function	Opioids prescribed solely for pain relief rarely result in addiction. The level of risk is not known, but many studies have shown it to be small
Dose restrictions	The smallest possible dose must be used, up to a stipulated maximum dose for each opioid	There are no specified maximum doses for opioids. For each individual the doses of regular and breakthrough opioid should be titrated to the level of pain
Opioid diversion	Prescribers are reluctant to issue prescriptions in case the opioid is diverted to someone other than the patient for inappropriate use	Healthcare professionals should always be aware of this potential risk and make efforts to prevent diversion. It should not interfere with rational and appropriate opioid prescribing for pain
Physical dependence	Opioids should not be prescribed in case patients become physically dependent on them leading to withdrawal symptoms when the opioid is abruptly stopped	Physical dependence is common in patients on a stable opioid dose. But it is not important clinically if opioid doses are reduced gradually before stopping treatment
Psychological dependence	Patients develop a compulsion to use the opioid	Psychological dependence is rarely seen in patients who are on a stable dose of opioid for pain
Respiratory depression	Respiratory depression limits the doses of opioids	When opioid doses are carefully titrated it is not a problem
Tolerance	Once a patient commences opioid treatment the dose will have to be increased frequently to overcome tolerance	Tolerance to opioids in chronic pain patients is uncommon. Titration of doses to achieve optimum pain control may take several months but the majority of patients are eventually stabilized on a long-term dose

Adverse effects

Opioid analgesics share many side effects, although each individual opioid has its own idiosyncrasies. There is rarely any advantage in choosing another opioid in preference to morphine unless it has a specific therapeutic benefit or pharmaceutical benefit. An example is the use of diamorphine, which has better water solubility than morphine, making it more versatile when delivered subcutaneously in palliative care, and epidurally in postoperative pain.

Morphine dosing

Morphine is the most valuable opioid analgesic for all forms of severe pain. It is the standard against which other analgesics are compared. It is available in a range of formulations enabling its administration by a number of different routes. The main therapeutic effects of morphine are sedation, mental relaxation and euphoria in addition to analgesia. Its mood-elevating effect often reduces the patient's anxiety about their pain.

When commencing a patient on morphine, immediate-release tablets are the most appropriate formulation. The starting dose should be 5–10 mg every 4 hours. It may be necessary to double the dose every 24 hours until good pain relief is achieved. Once the patient's dose has been stabilized the total number of milligrams of morphine taken in 24 hours can be divided by two and given as modified-release morphine tablets or capsules every 12 hours. The patient must continue to have access to immediate release morphine to take for relief of breakthrough pain.

If, after several days, it is found that frequent breakthrough dosing is necessary then the total daily morphine intake should be recalculated and divided by two to give the new dose of modified-release morphine. This titration process should be continued until stable dosing and effective pain control are achieved. This method is feasible in a hospital inpatient setting. For domiciliary patients newly converted to morphine it is normal to commence with a modified-release preparation of 20–30 mg every 12 hours, accompanied by an immediate-release preparation for breakthrough pain of 5–10 mg 3–4-hourly when needed, with review after 1–2 weeks. Tablets and capsules are the easiest formulations to use for the majority of patients. Oral morphine solutions (immediate release) and granules (modified release) can be used in patients with swallowing problems.

Preparations

The majority of modified release properties allow morphine to be active for 12 hours. At least one brand has 24-hour activity. Although a single daily dose is intended to make administration easier for the patient, in practice 12-hour release preparations are preferred.

Availability

All morphine sulphate preparations are controlled drugs and are available only on prescription.

Other strong opioids used in chronic pain

Diamorphine (heroin) is a slightly more potent analgesic than morphine. It may cause less nausea and hypotension. When given by injection it is partly converted to morphine. Its greater solubility in water allows the use of stronger injectable preparations than morphine. It is less lipid soluble than morphine, making it the preferred opioid for epidural administration.

Diamorphine injection is a controlled drug and is available only on prescription. It is widely used in the UK but is not available in many European countries nor in the USA.

Fentanyl is an opioid analgesic that is popular in general anaesthesia. It is 50–100 times more potent than morphine. It is sometimes combined with the local anaesthetic bupivacaine in epidural analgesia. A skin patch, described as a transdermal formulation, containing fentanyl is indicated for use in chronic pain. The patient applies a patch to a hairless area on the chest wall and leaves it for 3 days before removing it and applying a new patch to an adjacent area. Different strengths are available so that the dose can be titrated to the degree of pain. More than one patch may be used at a time for doses greater than 100 μg/h.

Patches do not suit all patients. Adherence to the skin for 3 days can be difficult. The 72-hour release properties of the patch are sometimes questioned, and the absorption of any medicine through the skin is a variable process. If severe side effects do occur that warrant patch removal the patient should be monitored for the next 24 hours. Fentanyl already in the skin will continue to be absorbed into the bloodstream. It can take 17 hours or more for the plasma fentanyl concentration to reduce by 50%.

Fentanyl patches '25' (releasing approximately 25 μg/h for 72 hours), '50', '75' and '100' are available only on prescription.

Oxycodone is a strong opioid that has similar properties to, but is slightly more potent than, morphine. Trials suggest that 1mg oxycodone is as effective as 1.5 mg morphine. It has been available for decades in the UK in the form of suppositories, but more recently has been made available in modified- and immediate-release oral formulations. An injectable preparation is also available. It is primarily being promoted for palliative care, although it is an alternative to morphine in chronic pain.

Oxycodone has the usual opioid side effects including constipation, sedation, nausea, vomiting and pruritis (itching). Some studies in chronic cancer-related pain have found that modified-release oxycodone resulted in less itching than morphine and no hallucinations. Other studies recommend the use of oxycodone in preference to morphine in patients with renal impairment.

Novel methods for delivery of strong opioids – intrathecal pumps

Syringe drivers are frequently used for the administration of diamorphine and other medicines into subcutaneous tissue in the end stages of life in palliative care. The subcutaneous route is inconvenient for the long-term relief of chronic pain. Some patients who experience unacceptable side effects from oral opioids respond well to the much smaller doses that can be delivered directly into the spinal cord. This invasive technique requires complex technical support and can be subject to a range of complications and adverse effects. The availability of an adequately resourced multidisciplinary team is essential to support the use of intrathecal pumps. The marked improvement in the quality of life of some patients prepared to take the risks is a strong influence on those pain specialists who are prepared to learn and develop the skills required for the safe use of this route. A comprehensive review of the many issues involved in using this mode of medicines administration was published in 2000 as a Health Technology Assessment by the United Kingdom National Health Service Research and Development Team (Williams et al., 2000)

In the 1970s the existence of opioid receptors in the spinal cord was demonstrated. Subsequently it was shown that opioids administered into the epidural space produced analgesic effects by being absorbed directly into the spinal cord and cerebrospinal fluid. The doses required to produce effective analgesia by this route are minute compared to doses given by other routes: 300 mg morphine *by mouth* is approximately equivalent to 10 mg morphine *epidurally* or 1 mg morphine *intrathecally*.

Delivering morphine or another opioid directly to receptors in the spinal cord avoids the problems of absorption, so requiring smaller doses. This in turn results in a reduced incidence of side effects.

Specialized pump systems have been developed for the long-term infusion of intrathecal opioids. The most technically advanced pumps are implanted under the skin of the patient's chest or abdominal wall. An implanted catheter runs from the pump to the site of entry in the intrathecal space. An internal battery with a life of several years drives the pump. The rate of infusion can be adjusted externally using telemetry. The opioid solution is held in a reservoir within the pump. It can be refilled by injecting through a port just beneath the skin.

Morphine is the opioid solution most commonly used in these pumps. All solutions infused intrathecally (and epidurally) must be preservative free. Unpreserved injections of morphine sulphate can be obtained from specialist pharmaceutical manufacturers. Limitations of using morphine in these pumps include:

- the highest strength available is morphine sulphate 40 mg in 1 ml;
- one pump model in current use has a reservoir volume of 18 ml;

- by filling this with morphine sulphate 40 mg/ml the maximum amount it can contain is $40 \times 18 = 720$ mg morphine;
- for a pump set to deliver 8 mg over 24 hours this reservoir will last $720 \div 8 = 90$ days;
- increasing the daily dose of morphine shortens the refill interval.

For the occasional patient with very high opioid requirements the refill period becomes so frequent that it inconveniences both the patient and the pain specialists. Strategies to overcome this include adding in a second pharmacological agent that allows a reduction in opioid requirements. Clonidine, an alpha-receptor agonist, and bupivacaine, a local anaesthetic, are two such agents. Alternative opioids to morphine can be useful in some patients. Diamorphine is no longer an option with some types of pump. Oxycodone is being evaluated to determine its usefulness.

Preparations

Bupivicaine injection 2.5 mg/ml (0.25%), 5 mg/ml (0.5%). These standard concentrations of bupivacaine are generally too weak for use in intrathecal pumps.

Bupivicaine injection 30mg/ml (3%) can be obtained from some specialist hospital pharmacy sterile manufacturing units as an unlicensed special.

Clonidine injection 150 µg/ml is available as a licensed preparation for hypertension. This weak strength has limited use in intrathecal pumps.

Clonidine injection 2 mg/ml (2000 µg/ml) can be obtained from specialist hospital pharmacy sterile manufacturing units as an unlicensed special. Bupivacaine and clonidine are prescription-only medicines (POM).

Pharmaceutical issues

There are many pharmaceutical issues involved in the safe use of implantable intrathecal pumps. These can be split into microbiological factors and physico-chemical factors.

With regard to microbiological factors, the solutions used must be completely sterile, and manipulated and administered using a strict aseptic technique. The solution may be held in the pump reservoir at body temperature for up to 3 months. The solutions cannot contain preservatives as these cause cerebral irritation. Any breakdown in aseptic technique may lead to bacteria entering the cerebrospinal fluid with consequent meningitis.

If solutions have to be reconstituted or mixed this should be performed in the strictly controlled conditions of a pharmacy aseptic unit. When combinations of analgesic medicines are used these are specifically tailored to the needs of each patient. Details of the amounts of each component solution must be recorded, plus their batch number and expiry date. The drawing up of solutions for intrathecal pumps at the patient bedside, whether this is in a theatre setting or an outpatient clinic carries enormous risks which can be lessened by using a licensed pharmacy aseptic facility.

With regard to physico-chemical factors, solutions of morphine sulphate are known to be stable for several months when stored at room temperature, but is its chemical breakdown accelerated when the solution is stored in a pump at room temperature? Undoubtedly it is, but analysis of residual morphine solutions removed from pumps in use show that there are still significant amounts of active morphine present at least 3 months after insertion into the pump. Solutions are generally considered 'stable' if there is still at least 90% of the analysed medicine present when it is reanalysed after a period of storage.

But how stable are solutions of morphine in the pump when another substance such as clonidine is added? Fortunately there is increasing evidence to demonstrate the physico-chemical safety of such combinations. A study examined the long-term stability in vitro of two concentrations of this combination and determined that the solutions were stable in the SynchroMed pump for at least 90 days at 37°C (Hildebrand et al., 2003).

Diamorphine and clonidine combinations were administered to hundreds of patients worldwide without apparent risk until reports of malfunctioning pumps appeared. An insoluble breakdown product of diamorphine is thought to be responsible for stalling the pump motor. In October 2003 the UK Medicines and Healthcare products Regulatory Agency (MHRA) issued a medical device alert (MDA/2003/035) stating that diamorphine should no longer be used in SynchroMed implantable pumps.

This emphasizes that, as well as establishing that analgesic combinations can be safely mixed together for long periods at 37°C, it is also essential to confirm that nothing put into the pump will interact dangerously with any material used in the manufacture of the pump or catheter.

A great deal more research is required to demonstrate the safety of medicines, especially combinations, in intrathecal pumps. This is particularly important given that the medicines are infused into the cerebrospinal fluid at very low flow rates from a reservoir that is refilled at intervals of between 4 and 12 weeks. Any interaction between medicines that results in chemical precipitation may have dire consequences for the patient.

Patient selection for intrathecal pumps

Such an invasive, risky and expensive method of analgesia is reserved for patients known to respond to large doses of opioids given by mouth but who cannot tolerate the associated side effects. Will the patient respond to intrathecal opioids? To determine the response to centrally administered opioids patients are trialled with morphine administered epidurally for a few days or weeks, and patient response is evaluated, if necessary, to increasing doses. Those patients who do obtain good pain relief can then be considered for an implantable intrathecal pump.

Adjuvant analgesics used in the management of chronic pain

An adjuvant is a substance included in a prescription to aid the action of other drugs (Roper, 1973). Many other medicine types can be used in chronic pain. These do not fall within defined steps on the pain ladder but can have a place at any point on the ladder for specific types of pain. They can be categorized as:

- topical NSAIDs;
- topical capsaicin;
- anticonvulsants;
- antidepressants;
- clonidine;
- cannabinoids.

Topical NSAIDs

Oral NSAIDs frequently cause side effects such as gastrointestinal bleeding, ulceration and occasionally perforation. To avoid these side effects pharmaceutical manufacturers have developed cream and gel NSAID formulations that are applied directly to the skin at the site of the pain source. Incidence of side effects from these topical preparations is small, such that restrictions on the availability of some NSAIDs in this form have been relaxed to allow them to be purchased 'over the counter' (OTC) from registered pharmacies.

Do they work or are they are expensive placebos? Initial scepticism about their usefulness has been moderated by reviews of the evidence. In patients with single joint arthritis or a rheumatological problem a topical NSAID gave effective pain relief and did not cause serious side effects. Some studies have shown the topical route to be as effective as the oral route. Reviews of the evidence can be found on the Oxford Pain website (see Further Reading).

Topical NSAIDs can be useful in chronic pain arising from specific points close to the skin surface. They are an option for a patient unable to tolerate oral NSAIDs but their use combined with oral NSAIDs is illogical and wasteful.

Topical capsaicin

Capsaicin is extracted from chillies. It is believed to deplete a chemical transmitter known as substance P that is found at nerve endings. Substance P plays some part in the start and continuation of pain processes. It has been implicated in a number of diseases including arthritis, psoriasis and inflammatory bowel disease.

Capsaicin is available as a cream. When applied to the skin it can be helpful in alleviating pain associated with diabetic neuropathy, osteoarthritis and psoriasis. It is not so useful in chronic pain associated either with postherpetic neuralgia or postmastectomy. It should be carefully applied to the local area affected. Its main side effect is skin irritation. Users are advised to avoid taking a hot shower or bath just before or just after applying capsaicin as this can worsen the burning sensation. This burning sensation may occur during initial treatment, particularly if too much cream is used or if the frequency of application is more than the recommended three to four times a day. This side effect may wear off with repeated use.

Axsain is a cream containing 0.075% capsaicin that is licensed for two indications:

* postherpetic neuralgia (after lesions have healed);
* painful diabetic neuropathy.

For both conditions it should be applied three to four times daily. Its use should be reviewed after 8 weeks. Zacin is a cream containing 0.025% capsaicin, which is licensed for symptomatic relief of osteoarthritis. A small amount should be applied four times a day.

Anticonvulsants

Some medicines commonly used in the management of epilepsy are useful in a variety of chronic pain syndromes. Anticonvulsants have for decades been part of the pain management of trigeminal neuralgia. They can be useful in managing the shooting pains associated with this condition and diabetic neuropathy. There is also increasing evidence of their usefulness in migraine prophylaxis and postherpetic neuralgia. They work by stabilizing nerve membranes to stop or slow down sporadic pain messages but their exact mechanism of action is unclear (Anon, 2000).

Carbamazepine can provide significant pain relief in trigeminal neuralgia. It is generally the treatment of choice for this condition. When taken during acute stages it can reduce the frequency and severity of attacks. Doses used range from 400 mg per day up to 2.4 g per day. Small doses should be used initially to reduce the incidence of side effects such as dizziness. Doses should then be increased slowly by 100–200 mg every 2 weeks. Blurring of vision, and unsteadiness in addition to dizziness often limit the dose. Use of modified-release preparations can reduce the incidence of side effects. Very rarely, carbamazepine causes agranulocytosis and aplastic anaemia. The manufacturers recommend monitoring of blood counts. Carbamazepine has been implicated in a number of drug interactions. Mostly these involve speeding up the liver metabolism of the interacting medicines, usually resulting in reduced effect.

Phenytoin has been tried in painful diabetic neuropathy. Some good results have been reported but in some studies it has not been significantly better than placebo.

Lamotrigine is a newer anticonvulsant. In addition to stabilizing nerve membranes it suppresses the release of glutamate from nerve endings. It can be effective in trigeminal neuralgia and painful diabetic neuropathy. In the latter condition it has been successfully used as an add-on with carbamazepine.

Gabapentin is a novel anticonvulsant with a mechanism that differs from those previously mentioned. It is licensed for the treatment of neuropathic pain, postherpetic neuralgia and trigeminal neuralgia.

Refer to the current edition of the *British National Formulary* or www.bnf.org for details of available anticonvulsant formulations. All anticonvulsants are prescription-only medicines.

Antidepressants

This class of medicines is effective in reducing neuropathic pain. Although they have been used for many years in the management of this type of pain, none of the many antidepressants sold in the UK is licensed for use in neuropathic pain.

Despite numerous studies there is no clear picture of whether antidepressants are superior to anticonvulsants. What is clear is that antidepressants have an effect on pain in addition to any effect on a patient's depressive condition. When used with opioids such as morphine they provide an analgesic effect.

Their use is limited by side effects. Thirty per cent of users can experience minor effects and up to 4% have to stop treatment because of the severity of the side effects. Sedation can be a beneficial side effect, giving patients better sleep.

Newer antidepressants such as the SSRIs include:

- citalopram;
- fluoxetine;
- paroxetine.

These have fewer side effects but have not be found to be as effective as the older, more 'dirty' tricyclic antidepressants such as:

- amitriptyline;
- imipramine;
- nortriptyline.

These older medicines act on a wider range of pain transmitter pathways than their newer selective counterparts.

Antidepressants take 10–14 days to have a noticeable effect on mood but are faster acting for pain relief. Effective doses are often lower than those used for depression. Conditions in which studies have shown that antidepressants have analgesic benefits include diabetic neuropathy, postherpetic neuralgia and atypical facial pain.

Refer to the current edition of the *British National Formulary* or www.bnf.org for details of available antidepressant formulations. All antidepressants are prescription-only medicines.

Clonidine

Clonidine stimulates α-adrenergic receptors of the sympathetic nervous system. In small doses it is used to prevent migraine. At higher oral doses it is used as an antihypertensive but has been replaced by newer blood pressure-lowering agents. Rebound hypertension can occur when clonidine is withdrawn or doses are missed.

Clonidine has an analgesic effect by inhibiting pain impulses when they pass through the spinal column. It works on different receptors to opioids and has additive effects on pain when given in conjunction with morphine. Morphine and clonidine combinations are infused intrathecally, sometimes epidurally. Other routes, because of the hypotensive effect of clonidine, rarely give this combination.

Cannabinoids

Cannabinoids are a group of chemicals found in cannabis plants. There are frequent claims in the media about their pain-relieving properties and there are many champions of the legalization of cannabis for medical purposes. The principal counterargument is that plant-derived medicines need standardization and rigorous clinical trials to evaluate them properly. Extensive research is being undertaken on purified cannabis extracts. The initial findings were inconclusive (Zajicek et al., 2003).

Research has previously demonstrated that humans possess cannabinoid receptors in the central and peripheral nervous system. The exact purpose of these receptors is unclear. However, animal testing has shown that cannabinoids have an analgesic effect and can help in neuropathic pain.

Nabilone is a chemically produced cannabinoid available in the UK that is licensed for use in nausea and vomiting caused by cytotoxic chemotherapy. It has been tried in some chronic pain conditions but side effects limit its usefulness. Cannabis is used socially for producing feelings of wellbeing so it is generally these euphoriant effects that are most troublesome when it is used for medicinal purposes.

Until the CAMS study ('cannabinoids for treatment of spasticity and other symptoms related to multiple sclerosis, a multicentre randomized placebo-controlled trial') (Zajicek et al., 2003) clinical trials undertaken on cannabinoids were small in number and mostly of poor quality, many being only single-dose studies. Trials have used several different cannabinoids. In chronic non-malignant pain, oral tetrahydrocannabinol (THC) has demonstrated a similar analgesic effect to oral codeine in patients with neuropathic pain and spasticity. Only THC improved the spasticity. Other work suggests that when cannabinoids are used with opioids they have an opioid-sparing effect, allowing smaller opioid doses to be used.

Adverse effects associated with cannabinoids are frequently reported in these trials; some are severe. The major side effect is depression of the central nervous system. Whereas small doses give rise to stimulant effects such as euphoria, larger doses have the opposite effect. Anxiety, panic attacks, acute psychosis and paranoia are generally dose related. Other reported side effects include dry mouth, blurred vision, palpitations, tachycardia and postural hypotension.

The CAMS study (Zajicek et al., 2003) found that two purified cannabis preparations did not give significant improvement in muscle spasticity scores. But there was objective improvement in mobility and pain. The trial medicines were generally well tolerated but the cannabis effects did unmask patients in the active treatment arms of the study. Despite the failure of this study to clarify the role of cannabinoids in chronic pain it remains an exciting area of research and the findings of other studies are awaited.

Further reading

See the Oxford Pain website at www.jr2.ox.uk/bandolier/booth/painpag/.

References

Anon (2000) Drug treatment of neuropathic pain. *Drug and Therapeutic Bulletin* 38(12): 89–93.

Hildebrand KH, Elsberry DD, Hassenbusch SJ et al. (2003) Stability and compatibility of morphine-clonidine admixtures in an implantable infusion system. Journal of Pain and Symptom Management 25; 464–71.

Roper N (1973) Dictionary for Nurses. Edinburgh: Churchill Livingstone.

Simpson KH (2004) Opioids for persistent non-cancer pain: recommendations for clinical practice. Editorial III. British Journal of Anaesthesia 92: 326–8.

Williams JE, Louw G, Towlerton G (2000) Intrathecal pumps for giving opioids in chronic pain: a systematic review. Health Technology Assessment 4(32): iii–iv, 1–55.

Zajicek J, Fox P, Sanders H et al. (2003) Cannabinoids for treatment of spasticity and other symptoms related to multiple sclerosis (CAMS study): multicentre randomised placebo-controlled trial. The Lancet 362: 1517–26.

CHAPTER ELEVEN

Complementary therapies

Val Ali

Aim

To provide an overview of complementary and alternative therapies and how they are being used for patients suffering chronic pain.

Objectives

By the end of this chapter the reader will:

- be aware of the government's classification of complementary therapies;
- understand the Alexander technique and its relationship to people suffering chronic pain;
- understand t'ai chi and chi kung and how to implement them within the National Health Service;
- understand acupuncture and its increasing popularity within chronic pain clinics;
- be aware of the different acupuncture practices available, and understand how they are being used and integrated into the NHS.

Introduction

A UK survey in 1993 showed that 33% of the population had used some form of complementary therapy and that more than 10% had consulted a complementary practitioner in the previous year (Rankin-Box, 2001). In the 10 years since, there has been a growth in the use of complementary and alternative medicine (CAM) by the general public and CAM is becoming more relevant to mainstream healthcare professionals. In 1997 the Prince of Wales' Foundation for Integrated Health was established to consider how orthodox medicine, complementary medicine and alternative therapies could be integrated to provide holistic, patient-centred healthcare, especially in areas such as chronic pain and rehabilitation.

Complementary therapies and the NHS

A substantial amount of complementary medicine is provided by conventional healthcare professionals within existing NHS services. A UK survey in 1995 showed that almost 40% of GPs offer access to complementary therapies for their NHS patients, over 70% of which were paid for by the NHS. In 1998 a survey of hospices revealed that more than 90% offered complementary therapies. Chronic pain clinics, oncology units and rehabilitation wards are currently the main providers for complementary therapies (Rankin-Box, 2001).

Classification of therapies

In 2000, the House of Lords Select Committee on Science and Technology classified the numerous therapies into three main groups:

1. The first main group includes professionally organized therapies. The therapies are often described as discrete systems of healthcare in their own right. The NHS, however, does not readily employ practitioners from this group, apart from a small percentage of acupuncturists. Chiropractors, osteopaths, homoeopaths and herbalists are often referred to as a possible treatment option by chronic pain clinics but are rarely available on the NHS. Acupuncture, however, is becoming increasingly more popular within both the NHS and the private sector.
2. The second group of therapies incorporates therapies that have a reasonable body of evidence but are not yet regulated nationally. However, they give comfort and support to many people and are being used to complement conventional care especially in chronic pain clinics. They are more readily available and accepted within the NHS. They include the Alexander technique, aromatherapy, reflexology, hypnotherapy, shiatsu, reiki and t'ai chi.
3. The third group of therapies has no apparent established body of Western evidence to support claims of efficacy. These therapies are split into two subgroups:
   - therapies that include long-established and traditional systems of healthcare such as Ayurvedic medicine and traditional Chinese medicine;

- therapies such as crystal therapy, iridology, radionics and kinesiology, which lack any credible Western evidence base.

It is well established that chronic pain should be treated using a multi-disciplinary approach and that complementary therapies play a large part in treating and supporting this group of patients (Shealy, 2002).

Alexander technique

The Alexander technique is popularly described as helping with posture and relaxation. Habits of misuse become ingrained into daily life and like any habits the person perpetuates them without thinking about it. Since misuse is something done unconsciously, the Alexander technique shows the person how to recognize and stop what they are doing, and how consciously to develop a way of supporting the body's weight and moving that is both natural and efficient, both relaxed and energized, like a child's.

Frederick Matthias Alexander, an Australian actor who suffered a recurring loss of voice, developed the Alexander technique around the turn of the twentieth century. By observing himself in a mirror he concluded that his loss of voice was due to the tense position in which he habitually held his head. By correcting the relationship of the head, neck and spine during activity, he solved the problem over a number of years. This marked the beginning of the Alexander technique.

The technique's benefits include:

- Improvement in balance and coordination, greater self-awareness, better presence, improved vocal function and reduced tension.
- It may alleviate chronic back pain or other joint, muscle or connective tissue problems, postural distortion, and digestive and breathing difficulties.
- Though not a psychotherapy or cure for psychological complaints, the Alexander technique can bring some psychological benefits such as greater self-confidence, reduced anxiety and an enhanced ability to cope with stress.

If people experience discomfort or pain they suspect that something is 'wrong', although they may not be able to tell what it is. It is difficult to notice and change imbalances of tension because they are with the person all the time, so they feel normal. People often stop feeling tensions that become part of their everyday lives and develop poor habits. A good example of this is that, when very stooped, tense people are asked to try to stand upright, they feel as though they are leaning backwards and about to fall.

Alexander called this 'faulty sensory appreciation' meaning that, with time, harmful habits cause us to have a distorted feeling of what we are doing with our bodies. Human movement is thought to be most fluent when the head leads and the spine follows. This new experience is practised repeatedly to create new motor pathways, improving proprioception and upright posture and leading to enhanced coordination and balance (Alexander, 1996).

The Alexander technique can be applied anywhere and at any time: at home, working in the office, at school, performing on stage, and during sports and leisure activities. Natural poise and balance soon become a way of life. Lessons last between 40 minutes and 60 minutes and, whereas a few lessons can make a difference, for continuing self-improvement and for patients suffering chronic conditions and pain a minimum of 20–30 lessons is recommended. A couch, mirror and various types of chairs are used to allow patients to practise improved posture and sitting.

Controlled trials have reported enhanced respiratory function in healthy volunteers, greater functional reach in elderly women, and improvements in performance and reduced anxiety in musical students following training in the Alexander technique (Dennis, 1995). An uncontrolled trial of a multidisciplinary programme for 67 chronic back-pain sufferers incorporating lessons in Alexander technique reported improvements in pain that persisted for 6 months (Ernst, 2002).

However, learning the technique requires commitment and a great deal of practice by the student. It is also important that the Alexander teacher is appropriately trained. The Society of Teachers of the Alexander Technique (STAT) was established in 1958. There are now well over 650 teaching members of the society in the UK and over 2000 worldwide. They typically come from a background of performing arts, dance, theatre and music or, more recently, physical or occupational therapy and massage. Certified teachers undergo at least 3 years of training on an approved course involving 1600 hours of training. Unfortunately, due to lack of resources, most pain clinics are only able to recommend the Alexander technique privately. However, as there is an increasing awareness of how beneficial the technique can be to patients suffering chronic pain, hopefully the number of teachers practising within the NHS will become more widespread.

T'ai chi ch'uan

'T'ai chi' is short for t'ai chi ch'uan and is the name given to the series of movements developed from a form of Chinese martial art created by

Chang San Feng (1247–1368). T'ai chi ch'uan is used to enhance mental and physical health by integrating relaxation, meditation, breathing and postural techniques, which help develop balance and harmonious movements (Ernst, 2002). The full system includes individual exercises, flowing sequences (or 'forms') both open handed and with various 'weapons', partner work and meditation. Because of the emphasis on developing and harmonizing internal structure, circulation and energy rather than muscular force, these arts can be practised by people of all ages, types and abilities, even those who might be prevented from joining in with other activities. They are commonly practised for stress relief, hypertension, good health and meditation or as martial arts, or any combination of these. Because of the many different aspects and approaches to these arts there are many different activities one can find in a class; some teachers will emphasize the martial aspect of t'ai chi, including various types of partner work, whereas others will concentrate on health aspects or teaching the basics, common to all aspects, like the long flowing forms that characterize t'ai chi. Some teachers will offer classes where the traditional forms and stances are adapted to specific needs (chronic pain), or integrate these into their more traditional classes.

T'ai chi ch'uan is normally taught in classes of 5–10 or more people. The atmosphere during practice is usually quiet, relaxed but intense. The student should maintain a level of concentration and should not be distracted by external influences. The group responding to advice and corrections by the teacher performs the movements simultaneously. T'ai chi is a lifelong endeavour and regular practice is essential to achieve beneficial effects. Evidence from randomized controlled trials (RCTs) suggests beneficial effects of this form as an intervention to maintain balance and strength and to reduce the risk of falls in elderly individuals (Lai et al., 1995; Wolfe et al., 1996; Wolfson et al., 1996; Ernst, 2002).

It is important to realize, however, that these arts, while being very gentle and engaging with the individual student in a very personal way, may also involve long periods of standing and the ability to follow sequences of movements. Many people find that they quickly learn the methods involved and benefit greatly from this; others, however, may find that the initial difficulties are too great for them to overcome and so drop out.

What are the benefits of t'ai chi for people suffering chronic pain?

- T'ai chi improves balance and coordination, strengthens circulation and respiration, and is a relaxing form of moving meditation.
- T'ai chi heals the mind, emotions, body and spirit.
- It can be practised indoors and out and can be easily incorporated into the day's routine.

These arts have long been practised in China as health aids; regardless of ability, simply engaging in these practices can help the student develop a calm and vibrant feeling of wellbeing. By working with an awareness of oneself an individual can start to improve posture, balance and mobility. Reducing stress and tension can help one work positively with mental and physical problems such as chronic pain and depression. Circulation, breathing, concentration and awareness can also be improved. Because of the emphasis on individual awareness of how the basic principles affect us these benefits can be, and are, enjoyed by a wide range of people of all ages and many different physical abilities.

What should an individual know before joining a class?

If health professionals are unsure whether a class is suitable for clients then they should talk to the teacher beforehand if at all possible. They should explain to the practitioner as clearly as possible what the person's particular needs are. Things that they might want to ask are:

- Do they have classes available that are more appropriate to the patients'/clients' needs?
- Will they be able to offer advice about how movements might be adapted to suit the patient/client?
- Are they willing to let the patient/client have a learning partner in the class with them should they require one?

The teacher should be more than happy to discuss these issues.

Finding a class

There are a growing number of people beginning to teach t'ai chi and many of these are electing to do so through community education colleges or private health centres. A teacher may be a part of a particular school or organization, but this may not always be the case; there are many good teachers working independently. The T'ai chi Forum for Health and Special Needs is aware of many teachers who are willing to adapt the traditional exercises.

What should one look for in a t'ai chi instructor?

- A good teacher must have been practising t'ai chi for at least 5 years before being given permission to think about teaching.
- They should have a good understanding of traditional Chinese medicine, and show knowledge of energy and t'ai chi healing postures (which posture is good for which complaint).

- They should have a pragmatic and realistic approach to the form, encouraging a gentle 70% approach at all times and not promising miracle cures.
- They should be able to show their instructor certification in a recognized school of t'ai chi and be a member of the T'ai Chi Union for Great Britain or the Chinese Martial Arts Association.
- It is doubtful that t'ai chi can cause actual harm but it can aggravate certain conditions. So the instructor should be able to display a reasonable understanding of contraindications for such things as diabetes and epilepsy.

The objectives of t'ai chi ch'uan for help in pain relief are:

- to reduce stress;
- mental relaxation;
- physical relaxation;
- improved physical balance;
- improved coordination;
- increased sensitivity and body awareness;
- improved breathing/lung capacity;
- increased range of motion and strength;
- improved posture;
- feeling of self-worth and personal control.

These objectives are achieved through the tai chi ch'uan form. Its slow movements create an awareness of oneself and one's surroundings. The slowness requires good coordination and balance. As a consequence, breathing slows and becomes deeper. The concentration required enables clients to relax and be 'where they are'. The straightness of the posture will help the spine to align and strengthen. On a non-physical note, the chi or energy increases its flow through the body, giving greater stamina and muscle tone. Internal organs are gently massaged by the movements and energized by the chi flow.

The teacher can check a client's:

- blood pressure;
- height;
- weight;
- body mass index;
- ability to stand on one foot for 5 seconds;
- ability to lift hands above the head;
- standing up from a chair without using the hands;
- ability to catch a tennis ball.

All of the above can be measured when a client starts t'ai chi and can then be reviewed at 3- to 6-monthly intervals to evaluate outcomes.

Chi kung (qi gong)

Chi kung or qi gong is an ancient Chinese form of energy exercises still widely practised in modern China to prevent and heal disease and create balance in the body, mind, emotions and spirit. In this self-healing system prescribed therapeutic postures are practised every day. Although about 2000 different styles exist in mainland China, chi kung can be organized into five main types: holding still postures, moving postures, breathing exercises, meditative practices and leading the chi energy through the body with the mind. There are many reasons for practising chi kung: as well as improving health and reducing stress it can be practised as a form of meditation and as an aid to self-development or spiritual development.

Chi kung practices increase or manipulate the chi in the body. Chi is viewed, in traditional Chinese thought, as a sort of universal energy. Things that are alive have chi. Things that are dead no longer have chi. The Chinese believe this force moves through your body along meridians and that the body stores chi in specific vessels (neither meridians nor chi vessels correspond to any physical organ). The Chinese consider t'ai chi to be a chi kung (qi gong) practice as well as a martial art.

Chi kung practices encompass 6000 years of Chinese history and tradition and are used for physical health and emotional stability. Whereas some practices are medicinal and scientific in nature, others have the goal of achieving enlightenment or immortality, or improving martial arts skills.

Many claims made by chi kung literature are of dubious value. However, clearly something is happening in at least some of the phenomena the Chinese attribute to chi. Acupuncture claims to heal by removing chi blockage through the mechanism of inserting needles at specific points in the human body. Chi kung practitioners have demonstrated, under controlled conditions, the ability to regulate breathing, body temperature and blood pressure at will. Some research demonstrates a weak correlation between changes in electric potential at acupuncture points. The claims of chi kung practitioners are currently under study at the National Institute for Health in Washington and in Japan.

T'ai chi is considered an excellent chi kung practice for improving health, emotional stability, and overall physical conditioning and martial arts skills. Traditional Chinese medicine teaches that if the meridians are blocked and chi cannot flow or if overall chi levels drop below some threshold value the body becomes vulnerable to disease and deterioration. The movements and controlled breathing in t'ai chi are believed to significantly increase overall chi levels in the body and to move the chi around the body in beneficial patterns (like blowing out a clogged fuel line with high pressure air).

For more information on the activities of the T'ai chi and Chi Kung Forum for Health and Special Needs see their website at www.taichiandspecialneeds.co.uk; e-mail them at forum@connectfree. co.uk, or write to the TCCKF, Box 163, 792 Wilmslow Rd, Manchester M20 6UG.

Acupuncture

Acupuncture is a form of therapy that involves the insertion of fine needles into selected points in the body. It is generally regarded as having origi- nated in China some 3000 years ago, although acupuncture-like techniques have developed independently in several other communities around the world. Indeed, the earliest indication of the use of such techniques comes from Europe and is revealed by the study of the Tyrolean ice man whose recently discovered remains date back over 5000 years. In the East, acupuncture grew up as an integral part of Chinese medicine within its framework of Chinese philosophy and it is still practised within this trad- itional framework today. However, there are increasing numbers of healthcare professionals throughout the world training in what has become known as Western medical acupuncture. This combines the prac- tice of acupuncture with Western medical theory, techniques and treatment (Filshie and Cummings, 1999).

How does acupuncture work?

Since the late 1970s, scientists in both the East and the West have been investigating how acupuncture works. In the Eastern world acupuncture works by using points situated on various meridians that run throughout the body, which act as channels for energy, called chi. In the Western world there now seems no doubt that some of acupuncture's beneficial effects are produced through stimulation of nerves at the site of needle insertion. This results in the release of endorphins within the nervous system. Endorphins are one group of the body's naturally occurring chemical mes- sengers, and are best known for their powerful pain-killing effects, but they have other less recognized functions such as boosting the immune system. Acupuncture has also been found to release various neurotransmitters, including opioid peptides and serotonin (Han and Terenius, 1982; Andersson and Lundenberg, 1995).

Several acupuncture points relate to what Western physicians call 'trig- ger points', tender spots which, when pressed, produce pain elsewhere in the body. The similarity in distribution of the meridian paths and the trig- ger-point pain patterns suggests that it was the recognition of these patterns by the ancient Chinese that led to the development of meridian theory. However, no evidence has been found to confirm the physical existence of chi or the meridians (Ernst, 2002).

Acupuncture is particularly useful for treating muscular aches and pains. If a tender point is found when pressed or reproduces pain or other symptoms it is very likely that acupuncture will effect a cure or give substantial benefit. If headaches are suffered, related tender points may be found in the muscles of the neck and shoulders. If pain is running down the arm, related tender points may be found in the muscles of the shoulder girdle and, if you have pain running down the leg, related tender points may be found in the muscles of the hip girdle (Berman et al., 1999; Filshie and Cummings, 1999).

Different approaches

Broadly speaking practitioners take either a Western medical approach or an Eastern traditional approach to the use of acupuncture. Doctors and other healthcare workers (specialist nurses, physiotherapists) who are trained in orthodox medicine use acupuncture as one of a number of therapies available to them and will make an orthodox diagnosis before deciding on which therapy to use. Practitioners who use the Eastern or traditional approach make an assessment based on the patient's condition and predisposing factors. Their personality is also explored in order to build up a comprehensive diagnosis in terms of energy disturbance of the body or a particular organ. The assessment may also include examination of the tongue, palpation of both wrists and abdomen, and search for tender sites (Ernst, 2002).

Acupuncture points

No matter which approach is used, needles will be inserted into selected acupuncture points. The steel needles are typically about 30 mm long, very fine (0.25 mm) and disposable. Needles are generally left in place for up to 20–30 minutes.

Some people are needle phobic, perhaps because of past experience with injections. Acupuncture needles are much finer than those used for injections, and the ends have a different shape; consequently, if acupuncture needles are inserted quickly through the skin, the needle may be advanced into deeper tissue, where the most frequent sensation is one of dullness or numbness. This is traditionally thought to represent 'energy' accumulating around the needle and indicates that it is probably correctly sited for optimal effect.

Course of treatment

Initially treatments are at weekly intervals. As relief is prolonged then the interval between treatments lengthens. Typically patients may receive 6–12 sessions. However, chronic conditions will often require more sessions and regular maintenance visits.

Auricular acupuncture

Ear acupuncture or auricular acupuncture can be useful for painful and non-painful conditions as an alternative to, or in addition to, body acupuncture and may be useful in the treatment of drug and nicotine dependence. However, present evidence suggests that acupuncture is no better than placebo for nicotine withdrawal or weight reduction (Ernst, 1997; White et al., 1999).

Clinical evidence and conclusion

The current evidence supports the concept that acupuncture has more than a placebo effect in some conditions (Ernst, 2002). Systematic reviews have shown acupuncture to be more effective than placebo for treatment of chemotherapy-induced nausea and vomiting, early postoperative nausea and vomiting in adults, and dental pain (Vickers, 1996; Ernst and White, 1998; Lee and Done, 1999). The evidence also suggests it has an effect on migraine but the quality of evidence is poor (Melchart et al., 1999). More chronic pain sufferers are experiencing complementary therapies by their own volition and anecdotal evidence from self reports highlights they have a place in managing patients with chronic pain.

References

Andersson S, Lundenberg T (1995) Acupuncture from empiricism to science: functional background to acupuncture effects in pain and disease. Medical Hypotheses 45: 271–81.

Alexander FM (1996) The Use of the Self. London: Gollancz.

Berman BM, Ezzo J, Hadhazy V et al. (1999) Is acupuncture effective in the treatment of fibromyalgia? Journal of Family Practice 48: 213–18.

Dennis RJ (1995) Functional reach improvement in normal older women after Alexander technique instruction on music performance in high and low stress situations. Psychology and Music 23: 129–41.

Ernst E (1997) Acupuncture/acupressure for weight reduction? A systematic review. Wiener Klinische Wochenschrift 109: 60–2.

Ernst E (2002) The Desktop Guide to Complementary and Alternative Medicine. London: Mosby.

Ernst E, White AR (1998) Acupuncture for back pain: a meta analysis of randomized controlled trials. Archives of Internal Medicine 158: 2235–41.

Filshie J, Cummings TM (1999) Western Medical Acupuncture: A scientific appraisal. Oxford: Butterworth Heinemann, pp. 31–59.

Han J, Terenius L (1982) Neurochemical basis of acupuncture analgesia. Annual Review of Pharmacology and Toxicology 22: 193–220.

Lai J-S, Lan C, Wong M-K et al. (1995) Two year trends in cardiorespiratory function among older t'ai chi ch'uan practitioners and sedentary subjects. Journal of the American Geriatrics Society 43: 1222–7.

Lee A, Done ML (1999) The use of nonpharmacologic techniques to prevent postoperative nausea and vomiting: a meta-analysis. Anesthesia and Analgesia 88: 1362–9.

Melchart D, Linde K, Fischer P et al. (1999) Acupuncture for recurrent headaches: a systematic review of randomized controlled trials. Cephalagia 19: 779–86.

Rankin-Box D (2001) The Nurses' Handbook of Complementary Therapies, 2nd edn. London: Baillière Tindall.

Shealy NC (2002) The Directory of Complementary Therapies. London: Time-Life Books.

Vickers A (1996) Can acupuncture have specific effects on health? A systematic review of antiemesis trials. Journal of the Royal Society of Medicine 89: 303–11.

White A, Rampes H, Ernst E (1999) Acupuncture for Smoking Cessation. Oxford: Cochrane Library.

White AR, Resch KL, Ernst E (1999) A meta-analysis of acupuncture technique for smoking cessation. Tobacco Control 8(4): 393–7.

Wolf SL, Barnhart HX, Kutner NG et al. (1996) Reducing frailty and falls in older persons; an investigation of t'ai chi and computerised balance training. Journal of the American Geriatrics Society 44: 489–97.

Wolfson L, Whipple R, Derby C et al. (1996) Balance and strength in older adults: intervention gains and t'ai chi maintenance. Journal of the American Geriatrics Society 44: 498–506.

Index

Page numbers in **bold** type refer to figures; those in *italics* to tables. Page numbers marked with an asterisk (*) refer to tables which include details of uses, doses, frequency, side effects and formulation for the medicines concerned.

abdominal pain 69
absorption, of medicines 230–1
acetaminophen, *see* paracetamol
acetylcholine 51–2
acetylsalicylic acid, *see* aspirin
activity, *see* exercise
acupuncture 259, 265, 266–8
adhesions 193
adjuvant analgesics 252
adrenaline (epinephrine) 54
aerobic fitness 200–2
  exercise parameters 201–2
  therapeutic effects of 201
age 95
agonists 233
Alexander technique 260–1
allodynia 47, 49, 59
alternative therapies, *see* complementary
  therapies
amino acids 62
γ-aminobutyronic acid (GABA) 58
amitriptyline 232, 255
anaesthesia, *see* local anaesthetic agents
analgesia
  age and 95
  gender and 95
  sites of action **72**
  when cause of pain is known 119–20
  see also analgesics; *and individual*
    analgesics
analgesic effects
  of cold therapy 216
  of heat treatment 212
  of massage 220

analgesics 235–52
  adjuvant 252
  justifying choice of 117–18
  mild pain **235**, 235–9
  moderate pain **235**, 240–2
  nurses' lack of knowledge about 101
  severe pain **235**, 242–52
  WHO analgesic ladder 235
  see also analgesia; opioids; *and*
    individual analgesics
angina, refractory 146–7
angiotensin-converting enzyme (ACE)
  inhibitors 239
angiotensin II antagonists 239
antagonists 233
anti-epileptics, aspirin and 236
anticoagulants, aspirin and 236
anticonvulsants 253–4
antidepressants 239, 254–5
  with opioids 254
  tricyclic 255
anxiety 96–7, 157, 164
  and exercise 201
  and pain behaviour 187
appraisal of pain 102–7
  see also assessment of pain
articular cartilage
  deconditioning 193
  reconditioning 194
aspirin (acetylsalicylic acid) 236, *237, 238
  drug interactions 236
assessment of pain
  assessment tools 104–7, 125
  chronic pain 103–4

key factors 104
nurse's *v.* patient's 99
psychological, *see* psychological
    assessment
association, learning through 13
attention diversion 23
attitudes
  helpful 86–7
  unhelpful 83–6
autogenics 170
autonomic nervous system reflexes **50**,
    52–3
avoidance behaviour 187, 188, 189, 190–1
avoidance learning 13
Axsain 253

back pain 132–3, 146, 188–9, 191, 227–8
  physiological generators of pain
      perception 133
barriers
  definition 114
  to effective pain management 113–28
behaviour 16
  ABC of 13
  avoidance behaviour 187, 188, 189, 190–1
  behavioural advice 190–1
  behavioural management 12
  pain behaviours 7, 14–15
  planned 205
  routes of learning 13
  see also cognitive–behavioural model
beliefs about pain 20
biofeedback 21
biomedical diagnosis 189
biopsychosocial explanations of pain 7–8,
    10–11, 31
biopsychosocial model 8–11, 15, 18, 27, 31
body, as an obstruction 78–9
bones
  deconditioning 192
  reconditioning 194
breathing
  diaphragmatic 169
  script for 179–80
  stretching and 197
  see also respiratory system
Brief Pain Inventory (BPI) 106
bupivacaine 248, 250
buprenorphine 233, 244

callisthenics 199
CAMS study 256
candesartan 239
cannabinoids 255–6
capsaicin, topical 253
carbamazepine 253–4
cardiorespiratory fitness, *see* aerobic
    fitness
cardiovascular fitness, *see* aerobic fitness
cardiovascular system
  adverse effects of morphine *245*
  deconditioning 193
  reconditioning 194
carers, professional, *see* healthcare
    professionals
cartilage, *see* articular cartilage
case conferences 163
case examples 8–10, 27–30
celecoxib *237*, 238, 239
central nervous system **40**, 43
  adverse effects of morphine *245*
central neuronal circuits, reorganization
    of 67–8
central summation theory 43
cerebrum **38, 41**, 57
chest pains 69
chi 265, 266
chi kung (qi gong) 265–6
chronic pain cycle 156–8
cingulate gyrus 40, **41**
cingulotomy 40
ciprofloxacin 239
circulation, massage and 219
citalopram 254
classical conditioning, learning through 13
clonidine 250, 255
  and diamorphine 251
  and morphine 251, 255
co-codamol 242
co-proxamol *241*, 242
Code of Professional Conduct, UKCC 115
codeine 240
codeine phosphate 240, *241*, 242
cognitive–behavioural model 12–18
cognitive errors 22–3
cognitive strategy training 24
cold therapy 215–19
  analgesic effects 216
  application methods 217–19

contraindications/precautions *218*
haemodynamic effects 215
indications for use 216–17
metabolic effects 215
neuromuscular effects 216
physiological effects 215–16
therapeutic effects 216–17
collagen 192–3, 219
communication 102
  PMP contribution to 167
  in PMP teams 172–3
compartmentalization 5–6
complementary therapies 258–69
  classification 259–60
  and the NHS 259
conditioning, classical, learning
  through 13
confrontation 187
connective tissue
  deconditioning 192–3
  reconditioning 194
continuity of care, breakdown in 116
control 24
  gaining 86–7
  individual's perception of 11
  lack of 80–1
  locus of 24
  perceived 167
convergence–projection theory 70–1
cool-down technique 197, *203*
coping 22, 23, 167
  strategies to improve 23
  styles 96
corticosteroids 138
  aspirin and 236
cortisol 54
counter-stimulation 76
COX (cyclo-oxygenase) enzymes **61**, 62,
  238–9
cultural influences 97–8, 159–60
cutaneous stimulation 210–29
cyclo-oxygenase (COX) enzymes **61**, 62,
  238–9

deconditioning 191–4
depression 97, 157–8, 164
  and exercise 201
dextropropoxyphene *241*, 242
diagnosis, biomedical 189

diamorphine (heroin) *243*, 247, 248,
  249, 250, 251
  and clonidine 251
diclofenac 234, *237*, 238, 239
dihydrocodeine 240, *241*
distraction 76, 166
distress and long-term pain 156–8
distribution, of medicines in
  bloodstream 231
diuretics, NSAIDs and 239
doctor–patient relationship 25–7
documentation 98–9
drug rounds 124–5
drugs
  controlled administration 125–6
  see also medicines; *and specific drugs and
    drug groups*

ectopic firing 66
education
  for healthcare professionals 99, 101–2
  in pain-management programmes
    165
effleurage (superficial stroking) 223
effusion, effect of cold therapy 217
elasticity 196
elastin 192, 193
elimination
  first-pass 234
  of medicines 232
enalapril 239
endurance 198, 199–200, 201
enkephalins 58
environment 17
epidural injection *136*, 140–1
epinephrine, *see* adrenaline
ethics 114–15
European Consensus Statement 149
excretion, of medicines 232
exercise 21, 167, 186–7
  aerobic fitness 200–2
  attitude to 205
  callisthenics 199
  cool-down 197, *203*
  goal setting 205–6
  isokinetic 199
  isometric 198, 199, 200
  isotonic 198, 199, 200
  pacing of activity 21, 87, 167, 207

planning 194–5
quotas 207
reconditioning 194–7
selection 203–4
specificity 206
training effect 206
see also strength; stretching; warm-up
exertion scales 202
explanation, levels of 3–18
extraversion 95–6
eyes, adverse effects of morphine 245

facet joint injection/denervation 136,
   141–2
failed back syndrome 146
family dynamics 25
family influences 159–60
fear avoidance 187, 188, 189, 190–1
feelings 16
fentanyl 248
   skin patches 234, 248
fibromyalgia 139
fight–flight–fright response 53
fight or flight response 168
flexibility 195
   effect of cold therapy 217
   effect of heat treatment 213
   effect of massage 221
   therapeutic effects of 195–6
   see also stretching
fluoxetine 239, 254
frictions (deep massage) 223
frontal lobe 40, 41

GABA (γ-aminobutyric acid) 58
gabapentin 254
gastrointestinal system, adverse effects of
   morphine 245
gate-control theory 11–12, 43–4, 130
   in pain-management programmes 19
   spinal cord stimulation 145
   suppression of pain 57–9
   TENS and 225
gender 95
generalization, empirical 3
glyceryl trinitrate 234
goal setting 167, 205–6
group work 19
guided imagery 169–70

healing, effect of heat treatment 213
healthcare professionals 116–21
   beliefs 188–9
   characteristics of 102
   education 99, 101–2
   fear of patient opioid addiction 36,
      118–19
   influences 188–9
   knowledge/assessment deficits 101, 115
   myths and misconceptions about pain
      116–17
   role in helping patients 90
   under-recognition of pain 100–2
   under-treatment of pain 113, 114, 115
   see also nurses
healthcare system 123–4
heat treatment, superficial 211–15, 228
   analgesic effects 212
   application methods 214
   contraindications/precautions 214
   haemodynamic effects 211–12
   indications for use 212–13
   metabolic effects 211
   physiological effects 211–12
   therapeutic effects 212–13
heroin, see diamorphine
homunculus 39, 40
hope 87–9
Hospital Anxiety and Depression (HAD)
   index 106
hospital environment 114, 121–2
hyperalgesia 44, 47, 49, 59, 212

ibuprofen 236, *237, 238, 239
illness, pictorial representation of 89
imagery 169–70, 190
   script for 180–3
imaginative inattention 23
imaginative transformation of context of
   pain 23
imaginative transformation of pain 23
imipramine 255
immobilization, see deconditioning
inactivity, see deconditioning
inattention, imaginative 23
inflammation
   effect of cold therapy 217
   effect of heat treatment 213
Initial Pain Assessment Tool 106

injury
    pain and 41–2
    time course 49, **50**
insensitivity to pain, congenital 54
interdisciplinary teams 173
intervertebral discs
    deconditioning 193
    reconditioning 194
intrathecal drug therapy
    drug administration *136*, 144, 147–8
    indications 148
    trial-screening tests 151
intrathecal pumps 249–50
    follow-up 152
    patient selection 251–2
    pharmaceutical issues 250–1
    preparations for 250
    pump safety 251
intravenous sympathectomy *136*
invasive techniques 129–54
    contraindications 137
    summary *136*
ischaemia 53, 145–6

ketamine 63
kinesiophobia 187
kneading 223
knowledge, pain knowledge deficits 101,
    115

lamotrigine 254
learned helplessness 80
learning
    avoidance 13
    operant 13
learning theory 12–13
leg pain 132–3, 146
    physiological generators of pain
        perception 133
life activities, alterations to 81–3
life experience, areas of 15–18
limbic system **38**, 40, **41**
listening, not being listened to 83–5
lithium 239
litigation 14, 158–9
local anaesthetic agents (LAs) 137
    epidural injection 140–1
locus of control 24
lumbar sympathectomy *136*, 143–4

McGill Pain Questionnaire 106
malingering 159
massage 219–24
    analgesic effects 220
    circulatory effects 219
    connective tissue effects 219–20
    contraindications/precautions *222*
    deep 223
    indications for use 220–2
    physiological effects 219–20
    self-massage 222–3
    therapeutic effects 220–2
medicines
    enteric coatings 231, 233, 236
    management 167
    modified-release 231, 233–4
    routes of administration 233–4
    see also pharmacokinetic processes; *and
        specific drugs and drug groups*
metabolites 232
metabolization 232
Misuse of Drugs Act 1971 242
models 3, 31
    biopsychosocial 8–11, 15, 18, 27, 31
    cognitive–behavioural 12–18
    medical 4–6
    see also gate-control theory
morphine 232, 242, *243*, 244
    adverse effects *245*
    antidepressants and 254
    availability 247
    and clonidine 251, 255
    dosing 247
    preparations 247
morphine sulphate 249–50, 251
multidisciplinary teams 173
muscle relaxation
    active/passive 170
    script for 183–5
muscle spasm
    effect of cold therapy 216
    effect of heat treatment 213
    effect of massage 220–1
muscles
    contractions 198–9
    deconditioning 192
    reconditioning 194
musculoskeletal deconditioning 192
myofascial pain 138

nabilone 256
nerve blocks 130, 133–6, *136*
  diagnostic blocks/interventions 134, *134*, 135
  outcome 135–6
  paravertebral *136*, 143–4
  peripheral *136*, 139–40
  spinal 140–1
  stellate ganglion *136*, 143
  sympathetic 134, *136*, 142–4
  therapeutic blocks/interventions 134, *134*, 135
  thoracic perivertebral 143
nerve lesions 65–7
neural blockade, *see* nerve blocks
neuroaugmentation techniques 144
neurokinin receptors 62–3
neuromas 65–6
neuromatrix theory 45, 67–8
neuromodulation, advanced 134, 144–5
  contraindications 145
  maintenance/follow-up 152
  patient/family education 150
  patient selection/screening 148–50
  phases 144–5, 148–52
  postoperative care 151–2
  trial-screening tests 150–1
neuronal circuits, central, reorganization of 67–8
neurons 56
neuropathic pain 65–8
neurophysiological deconditioning 194
neuroplasticity, central 63
neurosignature 67
nicoumalone 236
NMDA receptors 63–5
nociception
  normal state 47–9, *48*, 49–57
  sensitized state *48*, 49, 59–64
  suppressed state *48*, 49, 57–9
nociceptive system 38–9, 47–9
  responses elicited by **39**
nociceptors 51, 54–6
  A-fibre 55, 225
  C-fibre 55, 60–1, 225
  polymodal 56
non-compliance 116
non-maleficence 115

non-steroidal anti-inflammatory drugs (NSAIDs) 61–2, 236, *237*, 238–9
  topical 252
noradrenaline (norepinephrine) **53**, 54
norepinephrine, *see* noradrenaline
nortriptyline 255
NSAIDs (non-steroidal anti-inflammatory drugs) 61–2, 236, *237*, 238–9
  topical 252
nurse–patient relationship 122–3
nurses
  fear of patient opioid addiction 101, 118–19
  identifiable cause of pain 119–20
  inappropriate knowledge 101
  justification of choice of analgesic 117–18
  perception of patient's pain 116
  questioning patient's right to be pain free 120–1
  see also healthcare professionals

oedema
  effect of cold therapy 217
  effect of massage 223
operant learning 13
opioid receptors 244, 249
opioids
  adverse effects 246–7
  barriers to availability 116
  controlled administration 125–6
  dose titration 244
  fear of patient addiction 36, 101, 118–19
  intrathecal administration 147
  myths and misconceptions about 115
  safety, common misconceptions *246*
  strong 242–52
  weak 240
  withdrawal symptoms 244
opiophobia 118
opt-in schemes 160, 164, **177**
Oswestry Disability Index 106
oxycodone 234, *243*, 248, 250

pacing of activity 21, 87, 167, 207
pain
  acute 45–7, 93, *94*
  acute *v.* chronic 93, *94*

appraisal 102–7
assessment, *see* assessment of pain
behaviours 7, 14–15
biopsychosocial explanations 7–8,
    10–11, 31
causing harm? 157
characteristics *69*
chronic 2, 3–4, *46*, 47, 64, 93, *94*,
    103–4
components of 12
congenital insensitivity to 54
deep somatic 68–70
deep *v.* superficial *69*
definitions 37–8, 93, 118
describing 37–8
dimensions of 38–41
hidden gains from 158–9
idiopathic 3, 6
individual variations in 94–8
influence of meaning on 6
injury and 41–2
insensitivity, congenital, to 54
living with 76–7
multifaceted nature of 165, **166**
myofascial 138
myths and misconceptions about
    116–17
nature of 37–42, 93–4
neuropathic 65–8
normal 47–9
patients' expectation of 121–2
patients' right to be pain free? 120–1
physiological knowledge 42–5
physiological response to **37**
prior experience of 97
psychological explanations 6–7
recognition of 98–9
referred 41, 70–1
reorganized *48*
searching for a source 132–3
sensation of **39**, 54
sensitized *48*, 49, 59–64
as a subjective experience 174
sufferers' experiences of 75–91
superficial *v.* deep *69*
suppressed *48*, 49, 57–9
theories of 42–5
transient 45, *46*, 47–9
types of 45–9, 92–3

under-recognition of 99–102
under-reporting of 100
under-treatment of 113, 114, 115
understanding of 89–90
unrelieved, reasons for 115–16
visceral 68–70
see also nociception; nociceptive
    system; transmission pathways
Pain Audit Collection System (PACS) 106
Pain Coping Style Inventory 96
pain gate, *see* gate-control theory
pain management
    effective, barriers to 113–28
    multidisciplinary approach 18
pain-management clinics 130–1
pain-management programmes (PMPs)
    18–25
    aims 18–19
    case conferences 163
    cognitive errors 22–3
    content 19–20, 165–7
    control 24
    exclusion criteria 178
    family dynamics 25
    group work 19
    inclusion criteria 178
    intradisciplinary involvement 163–4
    medication management 167
    participant feedback 171–2
    psychologist role 164–5
    self-efficacy 24–5, 167, 204
    skills training 20
    structure 19–20
    team communication 172–3
    see also coping; exercise; relaxation; stress
pain relief
    from cold therapy 216
    false expectations of 83–4
    from heat treatment 212
    from massage 220
paracetamol (acetaminophen) 236–8,
    *237, 238
    codeine and 240
paroxetine 239, 254
patches 234
patients
    attitude 205
    contributing towards unrelieved pain
        115–16

expectation of pain 121–2
misconceptions 187–8
motivation to adopt self-management
  approach 204
not requesting improved standards
  121–2
right to be pain free? 120–1
self-management 204
see also sufferers
pattern theory 5–6, 43
peptides 62
peripheral vascular disease (PVD) 142–3
personality types 95–6
phantom sensations 41, 67–8
pharmacodynamics 230
receptor function 233
pharmacokinetic processes 230
absorption 230–1
distribution 231
elimination 232
excretion 232
first-pass elimination 234
pharmacological management 230–57
pharmacology, definition 230
phenytoin 236, 254
physical reactions 17
physiological generators of pain
  perception 133
physiology 36–74
evolution of knowledge 42–5
planned behaviour theory 205
plasticity 196
PMPs, see pain-management programmes
power 198, 199
Prince of Wales' Foundation for
  Integrated Health 258–9
professionals, see healthcare
  professionals; nurses
prognosis 189–90
proprioception 194
proprioceptive neuromuscular
  facilitation (PNF) 196
psychological assessment 160–1
aim 160
case conferences 163
onward referral 162–3
opt-in scheme 160, 164, **177**
outcome 161–3
preparation for 160–1

purpose 160
semi-structured interview format
  160
psychological perspectives 155–85
conditions needing specialist services
  171
explanations of pain 6–7
personality types 95–6
see also psychological assessment
psychologists, role in pain management
  programmes 164–5
psychosocial issues 133
punishment, learning through 13

qi gong (chi kung) 265–6
quinolones 239

reactivation 186–209
receptor blockers 233
reconditioning 194–7
referred pain 41, 70–1
reflexes
autonomic 52–4
motor **52**
nociceptive 50, **57**
somatic 50–2
sympathetic **39**, 52–4
withdrawal **39**, 50–2
reinforcement, learning through 13
relationships
doctor–patient 25–7
nurse–patient 122–3
relaxation 20–1
effect of heat treatment 213
effect of massage 221
environment 170–1
methods 169–71
scripts for 179–85
training 168–9
relaxation response 168
respiratory system
adverse effects of morphine *245*
deconditioning 193
see also breathing
responsibility, individual's perception of
  11
rest 190
ritualistic practice 124–5
rofecoxib *237*, 238, 239

sciatica 141
selective serotonin reuptake inhibitors
    (SSRIs) 239, 254–5
self, loss of 79–83
self-efficacy 24–5, 167, 204
self-esteem 81
    massage and 222
self-management 204
self-massage 222–3
self-reflection 166
self-treatment 210–29
sensations 39
    phantom 41, 67–8
sensitization *48*, 49, 59–64
    central 59, **60**, 62–4, 66
    peripheral 59, **60**, 60–2
skills training 20
skin, adverse effects of morphine
    245
sleep hygiene 167
somatization 23
somatosensory cortex 39–40
specificity, exercise programmes 206
specificity theory 5–6, 42–3
spinal cord stimulation (SCS) *136*, 144,
    145–7
    follow-up 152
    indications 146–7
    screening trial 151
spinal nerve blocks 140–1
stellate ganglion block *136*, 143
strength 198–200
    exercise techniques 200
    resistance 199
    therapeutic effects of 198
    types of 199–200
stress 22
stress inoculation training 22
stretching
    ballistic 196
    breathing and 197
    developmental 197
    static 196
    techniques 196–7
    types of 196
    warmth and 197
    see also flexibility
stroking, superficial 223
substance misuse 162–3

sufferers
    experiences of pain 75–91
    under-recognition of pain 99–100
    under-reporting of pain 100
    see also patients
suppression of pain *48*, 49, 57–9
    spinal modulation **58**
    supraspinal modulation **58**
surgery, see invasive techniques
sympathectomy, see intravenous
    sympathectomy; lumbar
    sympathectomy

T cells 12
t'ai chi ch'uan (t'ai chi) 261–4, 266
    benefits 262
    joining a class 263–4
    objectives 264
TENS, see transcutaneous electrical nerve
    stimulation
tetrahydrocannabinol (THC) 256
theory formation 3
thinking 16, 17
    cognitive errors in 22–3
    patterns 15
thoracic perivertebral block 143
tissue damage, effect of cold therapy 217
tramadol *241*, 242
transcutaneous electrical nerve stimula-
    tion (TENS) 224–7, 228
    in acute pain 225, *226*
    application 225–6
    in chronic pain 225, *226*
    contraindications/precautions *227*
    endogenous opioid activity 225
    high-frequency 224, 225
    indications for treatment 225, *226*
    low frequency 224–5
    pain suppression 58–9
    therapeutic effects 225
    treatment time 226
transduction 51
transmission pathways
    central 56–7
    pain inhibitory **58**, 59
    peripheral 54–6
treatment
    achieving success in 173–4
    categories 131

continuum 131, **132**
    provision of individual therapy 161–2
    self-treatment 210–29
    under-treatment of pain 113, 114, 115
trigger-point injection *136*, 138–9
trigger-point release 223
trigger points 266–7

valproate 236
verbalization 96

Wang–Baker scale 106
warfarin 236, 238, 239
warm-up 197, 200, 202–3
    physiological changes during 202–3
    therapeutic effects of 203

wind-up 62
Wolff's law 194
work
    importance of 158
    loss of 159
World Health Organization (WHO)
    analgesic ladder 235
    mild pain **235**, 235–9
    moderate pain **235**, 240–2
    severe pain **235**, 242–52

Zacin 253